IN A SPIRIT OF CARING

Understanding and Finding Meaning in the Doctor-Patient Relationship

Lynn D. Carlisle, D.D.S.

D1501227

KENDALL/HUNT PUBLISHING COMPANY
4050 Westmark Drive   Dubuque, Iowa 52002

Contents

Permissions

A Special Note

I have struggled with the pronoun issues of "he-she" and the use of the noun doctor-dentist in writing this book. I am very aware of the discrimination involved in the exclusive use of the masculine pronoun. The doctor-dentist issue is similar, but not as pronounced. I feel that there is no satisfactory solution to these problems.

I have chosen to use the masculine pronoun throughout the book. This choice is not an act of discrimination against the feminine perspective. The masculine pronoun is used because I feel the issues I write about in this book are historically masculine problems. This is because historically dentistry has been a male dominated profession. Many problems I address in the book derive from the masculine enculturation of dentistry. I think the women who have graduated from dental school experience the same problems. This is a result of spending four or more years in dental school.

The doctor-dentist and patient-client issues are not as clear cut. I hope my use of doctor or dentist and patient or client does not confuse the reader and detract from his or (her!) enjoyment of reading the book.

Preface

Dentistry is undergoing a period of profound change and transition in delivery systems and the core values of dentistry. Fear and anxiety are being manifested by many people in dentistry as time tested ways of practicing are no longer working. There has been talk of the end of dentistry's "golden era" of the 50's, 60's, 70's and early 80's.

There is no doubt that this era of dentistry is ending. The natural monopoly and sovereignty of dentistry is ending because of a higher ratio of dentists to population, increased productivity, a declining dental disease rate, a proliferation of delivery systems and an increasing number of governmental and private agencies that are attempting to manage and regulate dental care.

As this era of dentistry has been ending, a new way of practicing dentistry has been quietly emerging. This new model of health care grew out of the recognition by the pioneers in the preventive dentistry movement that in order to help patients prevent dental disease, a different model of health care needed to be developed. This new model was based upon the establishment of a helping relationship between the dentist and the patient. The intent of this relationship was to create a facilitative, caring and healing environment, in which the patient, dentist and team members would learn, grow, change and heal.

Many believe that this model will be a pacesetter for all of the health care professions in the coming years. Its focus on the patient, its respect for the patient's autonomy and its drive toward health and wholeness, provides an environment and level of care that is very rewarding for the patients AND for the dentists that have built their practices around this model.

The book explores a facilitative, caring doctor-patient relationship as the foundation to effective, humane health care; the contributions of preventive dentistry to learning how people learn; the need for a new model of health care. It addresses the dimensions of the helping relationship as it applies to the doctor-patient relationship; how people learn and grow; the importance of caring; the concept of the wounded healer; applications in the private practice setting; challenging and confronting patients; humanistic applications in dentistry; the importance of dentists taking care of themselves; and dentistry as a spiritual discipline.

The book is a combination of the author's own experience in integrating the human dimensions in his professional and personal life and research that has been done on helping relationships.

Acknowledgements

On first glances, writing a book is a solitary endeavor. The writer sits at a keyboard and composes a book. For me this is best done in a quiet environment without interruptions. This solitude is an illusion. I have been aware that there are people whose ideas have been with me during the writing of this book.

I want to acknowledge these people. It is very evident that the work and personhood of Carl Rogers and Art Combs were major influences in this book. Often, I was unsure whether the words I was writing were my own or were echoes of Rogers and Combs. I have tried to attribute their work appropriately. Art Combs has been an invaluable source of knowledge, inspiration and counseling. He has helped guide me as a first time author, through the maze of the writing and publishing business.

The L.D. Pankey Institute for Advanced Dental Education has played a pivotal role in my growth as a dentist. Loren Miller, John Anderson, Henry Tanner, Harold Wirth and L.D.Pankey helped me integrate the technical and philosophical sides of dentistry.

First Pacific Corporation of Portland, Oregon donated the hardware and software that I used in the preparation of the manuscript. I thank them.

I want to recognize another group of people in dentistry. They have been mentors and fellow travelers on my journey of understanding and developing person-centered approaches in my practice life. Wilson Southam's ideas and vision have been sources of inspiration for me. His ideas are especially evident in Chapter One, Six, Ten and Eleven. Avrom King's support, guidance and writings helped me, early in my dental career, to understand and implement the person-centered approach in my dental practice. Avrom awakened my interest in writing by publishing my Dr. Becoming letters in his newsletter, NEXUS. Omer Reed and Bob Barkley introduced me to the idea of humanistic approaches in dentistry.

Doug Young, Bud Ham, Bob Frazer, Cliff Katz, Judy Ham, Marlyn Young and Bruce Pettersen's ideas, friendship, understanding and support through the forum of the Bob Barkley Foundation are reflected throughout the book. I also want to acknowledge the dentists and team members I have interacted with in study group meetings and workshops I have attended and facilitated.

Gay Swenson, Arlene Wiltberger, Nel Kandel, Andre Auw and Janet Quinn have modeled and helped me learn about person-centered ways of being and learning.

And my family—my wife, Kirsten, my parents, Al and Gibby Carlisle, my brother Dick Carlisle and my co-workers, especially Jeanne Carnes. They have supported and helped me on my journey of becoming.

Last, I want to recognize my clients who have been my constant teachers with their opinions, criticism and support.

I hope that I honor these people and their influence on me by writing this book.

Introduction

There is very little, if anything, which I have written about in this book that is new. In researching this book I came across countless articles and books that addressed problems in health care similar to the ones I have addressed. So the ideas I have presented are at best "revolutionary old ideas." It seems that dentistry and health care have been addressing the same old problems since human beings first began to treat illness, trauma and disease. Yet, a reading of history shows that there are leaps of knowledge that occur in nonlinear ways. These leaps seem to occur spontaneously. They result from clusters of conditions spiraling together to demand new ways of dealing with problems. When a society recognizes the need for a new way of solving these problems, a paradigm shift occurs. Paradigm shifts, or changes in patterns, have gestation periods of several years to centuries. Paradigms are clusters of beliefs, attitudes and approaches that a culture (including scientific cultures) bases its values upon. A paradigm becomes a map to solving the society's problems.

A Paradigm Shift

It is my feeling that dentistry and health care are in the midst of a paradigm shift. The challenge dentistry faces is to bring along the valuable attributes of the old paradigm and to leave behind those that are no longer valuable. In the midst of these shifts, dentistry and health care have a chance to leave some seemingly timeless problems behind. It will require a change in thinking of doctors and clients.

The Paradox of Doctoring

Doctors will always be limited in their ability to treat trauma, illness and disease. It is the nature of the human condition that the potential for illness, injury, disease and death is always present for humans. Doctors will always make mistakes, not from malfeasance, but from their humanness. Doctors also paradoxically have the ability and training to perform seeming miracles. This paradox will never be resolved. The specifics will change; diseases will be mastered; surgical procedures will be perfected to return people to health; miracles will occur and still there will be failures and mistakes.

I believe that the attitudes that have occurred around the emphasis on science have been very valuable in the mechanics of health care. They have failed miserably in the human dimension of the doctor-patient relationship. "When strengths are over extended, they become weaknesses." The overextension of the attitudes of science—objectiveness, the body-mind split, distrust or ignorance of the nonphysical—has led health care away from the solid foundation created by a caring doctor-patient relationship.

Mechanistic science has been responsible for many advances in health care. The tendency has been to venerate the mechanistic or reductionistic method of science. Science is merely a tool to help understand the nature of things and to solve problems. The difficulty with veneration is the power and credence given to the subject of our veneration. This veneration leads to a failure to see science's shortcomings or the overextensions of its strengths. A doctor's focus needs to be on helping people to become healthier. Whatever helps him to do that is important. Science is one of those things, but it is just part of the kaleidoscope of tools that doctors use. Science loses its strength when it is venerated while other ways of helping people are discounted because they are not "scientific." Everything is scientific, if the definition of science as the process of discovering the nature of things and to solve problems is used. Mechanistic science is non scientific when it disparages, dismisses or discounts the validity of the human dimensions of health care.

I have a deep belief in the ability of people to grow and change. I have witnessed this ability in many people, particularly in my fellow dentists. It is not an easy process, and it is not for the faint of heart, but it is possible. Somehow, our institutions and systems in health care have become unhealthy for doctors, patients and other health care workers. These systems need change. However, systems change only after the people in the system change. To change a system, people first need to change in their heart and when enough people have changed, then the system will follow along. We will never have a perfect health care system. There will always be problems. Problems are the stuff of growth. They provide the grist for the mill of change.

Threshold of a Revolution

Dentistry is on the threshold of a revolution similar to the discovery of the germ theory. The revolution is the recognition of the role that the human dimensions of health care and our mind and spirit play in our health. The understanding and integration of caring doctor-patient relationships will transform the role of a doctor. These caring relationships, with patients or clients, will be the keystone to their success and enjoyment as a doctor.

What do I see as the results of this revolution and what implications does it have for dentists? The integration of the human dimensions in health care will help dentists to move:

+ from competition to cooperation among colleagues
+ from an orientation on money and technology to an emphasis on service and healing
+ from the agnostic to the spiritual
+ from the mechanistic to the humanistic
+ from complexity in doctors' lives to simplicity
+ from the reductionistic to the holistic
+ from burn out to enjoyment
+ from being a dispassionate expert to a caring collaborator
+ from hiding behind a facade to being genuine
+ from dissatisfaction to enjoyment of being a doctor

The writing of this book has been an enlightening process for me. I have been very aware that this process has been a classic case of the "teacher teaching what he most needs to learn." The topics I have written about in this book are challenging for me to learn.

It is my hope, that this book will help you start upon or enhance your journey toward feeling fulfilled in your practice of dentistry.

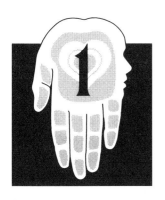

The End of an Era

When I first started practicing dentistry in 1968, I was amazed that my patients did not accept my recommendations for dental treatment. I had assumed that all I had to do was tell them what they needed and they would immediately schedule the treatment. After all I was a dentist, an expert in dental disease, and I knew what was best for them. When they did not accept the treatment I had recommended, I assumed that it was ignorance (or stupidity) on their part. It did not cross my mind that I was the one that was responsible for creating the problem.

As I look back, I realize that I was the naive and ignorant one. Fortunately for me, I became interested in the preventive dentistry movement that was beginning then. Preventive dentistry put dentistry in a different context for me. I taught patients disease control techniques and encouraged them to eat properly. However, I still had trouble motivating my patients to accept the treatment I felt they needed and to practice better oral hygiene. My frustration led to a search for the formula that would magically correct this problem.

Persistence is a strength and weakness of mine. So I persisted and kept looking for the magic answer. This search led to my fascination with how people learn and grow. It has enabled me to participate in dentistry's contribution of two of the most significant accomplishments in health care during the last 25 years. The first contribution is the reduction of two of humankind's three most common diseases—dental caries and periodontal disease (the common cold is the third). The second contribution is the development of a humanistic model of health care. This model includes the human dimensions of caring, respect and compassion, with the techniques of repair and prevention.

The Preventive Dentistry
Movement's Contributions

Both contributions originated in the preventive dentistry movement of 1965 to 1975. Since this time, the dental caries rate has dropped as much as 50% and in many children is non existent. Periodontal disease rates have also declined during that time.

The discovery in the late 1940's and early 1950's by C.C. Bass and Sumter Arnim of the importance of dental plaque removal in controlling dental disease, ranks with Ignaz Semmelweiss's great work on asepsis in the middle 1800's (and Harold Loe's work on experimental gingivitis and plaque in the middle sixties). Bob Barkley introduced their work on dental plaque to practicing dentists during the sixties and seventies. The work of these men along with the work of Weston Price, Royal Lee and Melvin Page's recognition of the importance of proper nutrition in preventing dental disease, laid the foundation for the preventive dentistry movement. (Frederick McKay's discovery of the role that fluoride plays in preventing dental caries was also a key factor in the reduction of dental caries.)

The work of these pioneers in preventing dental disease led to a dramatic reduction of dental disease. Practicing dentists used their findings to help their clients control their dental disease through proper dental plaque removal. This reduction of dental disease has become dentistry's greatest accomplishment, and I think is among the most important developments in health care in the last 20–30 years.

The following quotation reflects the significance of this accomplishment. The quotation is from an article written by Daniel S. Greenberg in the Boston Globe on March 29, 1987.

"Front page homage and reverence are heaped on organ transplants and other medical high-wire acts. Meanwhile dentistry goes unnoted, except as the butt of harebrained television humor. But, it is one of the few health technologies that almost invariably succeeds, both in prevention and in treatment. There is little else in the health care arsenal that can share that claim."

"Dentistry is one of the great success stories of our time. Viewed against the economic turmoil and limited achievements that generally afflict medical care, dentistry is especially notable for its advocacy of health education and public preventive measures."

A Humanistic Model of Health Care

The second contribution, a humanistic model of health care, evolved out of the efforts of a group of people in dentistry to help patients carry out the knowledge of what prevented dental disease. This knowledge of how to prevent dental disease created a need for a new delivery model of dental care. The following conclusions on the importance of facilitative relationships in dental practice are the result of a comprehensive study done in the early 1970's by the Illinois Academy of Dental Practice Administration, Bob Barkley, D.D.S. and psychologist Nathan Kohn Jr. Ph.D.:

> *"When a patient leaves your office able to explain to his friends his relationship with you and how it benefits him immediately and in the years ahead, you have established a relationship with that patient which is the only sound basis for growth of your practice and development of your profession."*

> *"Psychologists have discovered, as a matter of fact, that the inability of individual dentists, or the dental profession, to establish this relationship with patients is a major contributing factor to the problem of why more people do not avail themselves to adequate dental care."*

In the area of prevention, the patient's active participation in changing his lifestyle is the essential ingredient to improve his health. This placed different demands upon the doctor and patient and changed their relationship with each other. Previously, the patient was the passive dependent recipient of instructions and treatment by the doctor. The different demands resulted in a relationship based on the patient becoming an active interdependent member of a team devoted to helping him become well. The humanistic model was based upon helping patients learn new habits and health behavior as a foundation for any dental care or treatment that they needed. Bob Barkley wrote "As my philosophy of dental care matured, my self-image slowly changed from that of a 'healer' to an interested, empathic teacher of health who is also capable of good restorative dentistry."

The End of the "Golden Era"

Ironically, these two contributions seem to have led to the end of the era that some people have called "the golden age of dentistry" of the 50's, 60's, 70's and early 80's. The term golden era refers to a time when there was a high dental disease rate and not enough dentists to provide dental care.

Wilson Southam has written that the natural monopoly and sovereignty that dentistry enjoyed during this era have ended. Increased treatment productivity, a higher ratio of dentists to patients, declining dental disease rates, the proliferation of delivery systems, an increasing number of governmental and private agencies that are attempting to manage and regulate dental care, the closure of dental schools, a reduction in the size of dental schools classes and the public's wish to have a stronger voice in their health care, led to the end of this era.

In the face of the ending of this era, there is a tendency by many people in dentistry to hold on to the status quo and the past. They resist the changes that the end of this era of dentistry brings. It seems that the result of this ending of an era is the chaos that these changes are producing in dentistry. Dentistry is undergoing a period of profound change and transition in delivery systems and in the core values of dentistry. Yet out of these changes and seeming chaos there has been the quiet emergence of the humanistic model of health care.

New Model Is a Pacesetter in Health Care

Many people in dentistry believe that this new model will be the pacesetter for all of the health care professions in the coming years. Wilson Southam believes that the humanistic approaches focus on the patient; its respect for the patient's autonomy; its respect for the patient's drive toward health and wholeness provides an environment and level of care that is very rewarding for the patient and dental team. These dental teams are doing well both in terms of personal satisfaction and financial prosperity. Some practices are experiencing extraordinary success by any standard.

Dentistry is in a unique position in health care to be the leader in this new way of practicing. Dentistry's long experience with treating and preventing lifestyle related disease gives it a rich heritage to draw upon in helping other health care professions cope with lifestyle related diseases.

The foundation of this new model of dental care is helping clients make informed choices about their dental care. Facilitative communication by behaviorally skilled dentists and team members is the key to helping clients make these informed choices. Southam and John Stewart wrote that this way of practicing is built upon "The power in each of us to choose . . . to resolve . . . to will. In the context of health care delivery . . . to choose health . . . to resolve to take care of ourselves . . . to will the requisite new behaviors. — In a health care setting of authentic caring and freedom, most people will choose to strive toward higher levels of self care of their own volition."

Many names have been used in describing this new way of practicing. They include: relationship-based, health-centered, wellness-centered, values-based, person-centered, and Volitional Practice (tm). For the purposes of this book, person-centered will be used. The term person-centered was developed by Carl Rogers to emphasize that he felt the focus should be on the person being helped, and not the person doing the helping.

Unique Factors in Dentistry Led to the Development of This Model

There are some factors that are unique to dentistry that has led to its pioneering the development of the person-centered model.

✦ The pioneers in preventive dentistry recognized the importance of creating learning environments in the dental office to help people control dental disease. They recognized that learning involved more than lectures, instruction sheets or how to's. This discovery led to a search for how people learn and grow and the realization that the dentist's and team member's role was more than the mechanical treatment of disease. This search led to the work of Carl Rogers, Arthur Combs and others in humanistic psychology on the conditions that facilitate learning. Their work provided the theoretical basis for developing learning experiences to help dental patients control their dental disease.

✦ Dental diseases are lifestyle diseases. The correction or elimination of dental diseases is dependent upon the patient's commitment and active involvement in changing the risk factors that led to the disease. These risk factors include: nutritional imbalances, deficiencies or excesses, stress, lack of proper oral hygiene, psychological maladaptions, environmental toxins and social or societal dysfunctions. The recognition of these risk factors' role in dental disease led to an expanded awareness of the dentist's role as an educator and counselor. In this role, the dentist helped his patients change the lifestyles that led to the dental disease.

✦ The finest dentistry is discretionary. In the absence of swelling, bleeding or pain, dental work is discretionary. People choose to have discretionary dental treatment because of valuing high level health and well being and not just the elimination of the swelling, bleeding or pain. When people value their dental health, they choose to have dental work done to optimize their dental and general health and well being. When people do not value their dental health, they choose only what will get rid of the swelling, bleeding or pain. They do not look at the general relationship of their dental health to their well being. L.D. Pankey said that 90% of patients do not value and appreciate fine dentistry. He felt that they needed to be educated to value fine dentistry.

✦ Dentistry is not hospital based and usually does not incur the high cost associated with medical care. With rare exceptions, dentistry is not confronted with life threatening trauma or diseases and their associated high costs. People are generally well and healthy when they seek dental treatment. This permits a different set of dynamics of health care in dentistry.

Dentists have an opportunity to have interactions with people who can actively participate in the decisions for dental care. Technology is responsible for many of medicine's problems. These advances have broadened medicine's ability to diagnose and treat disease and trauma. Also, the rapid increase in technology has dehumanized the doctor/patient relationship. These advances are also significant factors in the rapid increase in medical costs. Major advances in dentistry have been in the prevention of dental disease, work simplification, ergonomic design of treatment areas and the usage of expanded duty auxiliaries. These advances have helped dentistry control the costs of dental care. Usually, people can be restored to maximum dental comfort and function at reasonable costs when compared to the cost of medical care.

✦ Dentistry does not deal (except in rare cases) with life threatening diseases. Dentists do not have to deal with the dynamics of death or terminal illnesses. Most patients that seek dental treatment are physically healthy. They can make sentient decisions with their full faculties. This provides the dental team with opportunities to build long term relationships. Without emergency or urgent care, the dental team can create learning environments to help the person learn to place a higher value on their dental health. Counseling patients to change destructive lifestyle habits and to incorporate wellness behaviors is also possible by dental teams. Time and urgency are removed as impediments to fine dental care. Without time and life urgency, the person can make voluntary, clarified, discretionary, value based decisions on when to have their dental work done. People can make long term plans for their dental health and general well being.

✦ Dentistry has been blessed with a group of people that could see the need for a new way of practicing dentistry. They have created the systems necessary to carry out the person-centered approach. These people include Bob Barkley, L.D. Pankey, Wilson Southam, Avrom King, Chuck Sorenson, Omer Reed, Doug Young, Bob Frazer, Cliff Katz, Bud Ham and Bruce Pettersen.

Philosophical Assumptions and Beliefs

All health care practitioners have a set of stated or unstated philosophical assumptions and beliefs. The decisions they make in the treatment of their patients are based upon these assumptions and beliefs. The following statements are the philosophical assumptions and beliefs of the person-centered approach to dentistry that have evolved over the years. Not every person or practice who uses the person-centered approach would subscribe to all of the listed assumptions and beliefs. The statements are clusters of assumptions and beliefs that most of the practitioners of the person-centered approach share. These assumptions and beliefs have been expanded upon for health care from Rogers' original premises.

Common characteristics or assumptions of the person-centered way of practicing dentistry are:

+ The patient is a respected equal and a partner or co-creator in the healing process, and is a responsible collaborator for his/her own health. The doctor is a facilitator, a resource, a partner with knowledge and skills to help the patient heal.
+ People have an innate drive toward health. They have within themselves the necessary ingredients, impulses and drives toward health and in an authentic facilitative climate will choose higher levels of health and wellness.
+ Illness is a disharmony of a person's physical, emotional and/or spiritual development. This disharmony impedes a person's growth and development. Illness and disease can be creative or generative. Illness and disease can lead to growth, change, development and new understandings by the patient.
+ Health is more than the absence of disease. Health includes the synergistic interaction of personal, social, interpersonal, societal, environmental, physical and spiritual factors. These factors do not exist in isolation from each other.
+ Human beings are each unique and can experience dynamic growth and change. Health and illness can lead to growth processes that result in integration and wholeness.
+ The personhood and genuineness of the doctor and team members are primary components of their care for the patient. Their attitudes and beliefs can either help or inhibit the healing of the patient.
+ The doctor is in the "business" of affirming life and supporting growth and changes in the persons who come for care. The doctor's and the patient's personhoods are primary components in healing. The person's life context is a factor in his illness or disease and contributes to his healing and well-being.
+ A dental team that is committed to the core values of the person-centered approach is essential to its application and to helping clients heal.
+ A caring doctor/team-patient relationship is the keystone to the success of the person-centered model. This relationship builds upon the belief that a respectful and compassionate caring with the intent to help the patient to grow and to heal, is foundational to dental care. This spirit of caring comes from the heart of the doctor and team. It provides the opportunity for the doctor and team to give of themselves and to feel fulfilled in their practice of dentistry.

The principles listed above, have created a need for new requirements for dentists to create a better model for nonurgent, primary health care. The person-centered model is based on the establishment of ongoing effective caring relationships; an understanding of how people grow and change; facilitating informed choice making; the application of humanistic behavioral approaches. Traditionally, dentistry is driven in its basic credibility by science, technology and technique. The person-centered approach believes that science, technology and techniques are part of a larger whole that includes the human dimensions of caring, respect and compassion. Besides dental treatment and prevention of dental disease, dentistry is in the behavior change and lifestyle business.

The person-centered model is challenging to carry out and to live. It involves: a personal clarification of personal and professional values, a knowledge of self and a recognition of one's strengths and weaknesses, a commitment to giving the best one has to offer, both technically and behaviorally, the intent to be fully present when helping clients heal, an openness to learn, grow and change, trust and belief in the patient's ability to heal, the development of a congruent philosophy of care, the development of a team whose actions and beliefs are congruent with the values of the person-centered model and the recognition of the importance of caring doctor/team-patient relationships.

Summary

So an era in dentistry has ended: an era in which dentistry moved from being a trade to being a profession, from placing fillings, removing teeth, and making dentures, to restoring the mouth to maximum comfort, function, health and esthetics through antibiotic therapy, surgical treatments, restorative techniques and orthodontic approaches. A new era is beginning. This new era includes the rich heritage of the old era. Also, it creates new, more humanistic ways of dental practice that includes the human dimensions of respect, caring and compassion for the patient. The foundation of this new approach is based on the establishment of effective helping relationships by the dental team and a caring relationship between the doctor and patient.

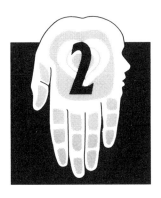

The Need for a New Model of Health Care

There are many people in dentistry who question the need for a new model of health care. They point to the accomplishments of dentistry and the medical model that led to these accomplishments and say, "Why change? Look at what the medical model has accomplished." These accomplishments resulted from the application of the scientific knowledge the medical model is based upon. The application of the scientific knowledge in the health care professions led to the development of technologies, drugs, instruments, tests and diagnostic approaches that helped the clinician's ability: to successfully diagnosis and treat most bacterial and viral infections, to treat the trauma such as the injuries that resulted from automobile accidents or athletic injuries, and to correct structural hereditary problems such as the orthodontic correction of malocclusions.

"Best of Times or Worst of Times?"

From this perspective it seems that these are the "best of times" in dentistry and the other health care professions. Dentists and other health care professionals have at their disposal more knowledge, more sophisticated techniques and better technology to help people return to health if they are ill or injured than at any other time in recorded history.

In health care, premature death due to the historical acute infectious disease in the United States is disappearing. Smallpox, mumps, measles, typhoid fever, diphtheria, tetanus and polio are almost nonexistent. Most people no longer know anyone who has these diseases. As mentioned in the previous chapter, dentistry's emphasis on prevention has led to the dramatic decrease in the incidence of dental caries and periodontal disease.

There are a wide array of techniques available to repair the damage to the mouth from traumatic injuries. The knowledge of the important role that proper nutrition, exercise and stress management has in a person's feeling of well being is being integrated into dental practices.

People's life spans are increasing. The U.S. Bureau of Health Statistics research shows that during the twentieth century, the life span from birth has increased from 47 to 75 years. The Office of the Actuary projects a life expectancy of 85 years by the year 2000.

Yet, in the midst of all these accomplishments, dentists are feeling besieged from all sides with demands that they do more, be more and give more, while receiving less fulfillment and compensation. An alphabet soup of businesses, insurance companies and governmental agencies are becoming wedges that are separating dentists from the touchstone of why they chose dentistry as a profession. That touchstone is to use their knowledge, caring and compassion to help people become healthier.

In a poll by Dental Economics magazine, over 50% of the 500+ respondents replied no to the question "If you had to do it over would you become a dentist again?" Dentists exist in an environment of their own and others' making that is increasingly complex, demanding and challenging. Dentists are feeling "burnt out," isolated, misunderstood and mistreated because of these demands.

The opportunity to serve people and the sense of prestige and fulfillment they sought in becoming a dentist has not appeared or has dissipated. In the midst of all the knowledge, techniques and technology there is something lacking. Like lost souls, dentists have lost touch with the human dimensions of dentistry; especially the caring doctor-patient relationship built upon a reciprocal compassion, caring and respect between the doctor and patient.

Six Pressing Reasons for Change

Dentists do care. They are compassionate. They are dedicated to helping their patients or clients become well. The lack of the human dimension for the dentist is not because he is lacking humaneness. It results from his lack of experience or training in how to manifest his humaneness. The need for reestablishing the human dimension is particularly pressing at this time. I believe it is pressing for the following reasons. (Fair or not, most governmental agencies, businesses, insurance companies and the public perceive dentistry as the same as medicine. The following reasons are presented, and therefore, I use some quotes that apply to medicine.)

1. The relationship between the doctor and patient is becoming an adversarial encounter. Time magazine in its July 31, 1989 cover story said "Doctor bashing has become a blood sport. — Small wonder that the doctor-patient relationship, once something of a sacred covenant, has been infected by the climate in which it grows." Another quotation from the Time magazine article is illustrative of the interference of third parties with the doctor-patient relationship. "The air of the operating room, where once the doctor was sovereign, is now so dense with the second guesses of insurers, regulators, lawyers, consultants and risk managers that the physician has little room to breathe, much less heal." Physicians and dentists are feeling a loss of control of their professional lives as these third parties attempt to manage health care decisions with interventions and regulations that endanger a caring doctor-patient relationship.

2. The public's perception of dentists and physicians is that they have been seduced by technology, money and specialization. They have little concern for patients and their questions, concerns, wants and needs.

3. The reductionistic scientific approach that prevails in and directs the values and beliefs of the health care system, needs to evolve into a more holistic approach that includes the emotional and spiritual dimensions of health care.

4. Counseling and communication is emphasized by the media, research and patients in dentist and physician interactions with patients. A report by the U.S. Preventive Services Task Force emphasized that to be more effective in preventing disease, dentists and physicians should spend more time counseling their patients on how to lead healthier lives through proper diet, exercise and other preventive means. The U.S. Department of Human Services commissioned a study to explore restructuring Medicaid reimbursement so counseling will be reimbursed at a higher rate while some surgical services reimbursements would be reduced.

A Wall Street Journal article titled "Sometimes Talk is the Best Medicine," quoted a research paper in the Maryland Medical Journal. "Poor communication between doctors and patients is the single most common cause of malpractice suits. — Health insurers increasingly believe that good doctor patient communication can avert malpractice suits and unnecessary surgery. A few underwriters already reward doctors who try to communicate better by reducing their malpractice premiums."

5. There is an increasing feeling of competition between doctors, as they believe there are not enough patients to go around. Instead of collegial relationships with fellow doctors, there is a feeling of rivalry and conflict as they scramble for patients.

6. Doctors and patients have lost their feeling of respect and reverence for the caring doctor-patient relationship's role in the healing process. Norman Cousins in *Human Options* stated this need well. "What is the most painful and devastating question that can be asked about modern medical practice? It is not whether most doctors are up to date in their knowledge or in their techniques, but whether too many know more about disease than about the person in whom the disease exists."

Chasm Between Doctor and Patient

What has led to the chasm between doctors and their patients and to the doctor "knowing more about disease than about the person in whom the disease exists"?

The origin of this attitude seems to have occurred in the mid to late 1800's as the discoveries of mechanistic or reductionistic science influenced the health care professions. Mechanistic science is based upon the work of Isaac Newton and Rene' Descartes. Mechanistic science's emphasis is on the body-mind split and the world as a very complex mechanical system. The image used in this approach is of a large complex cause-effect clockwork mechanism. Paul Starr wrote in *The Social Transformation of American Medicine*:

> "In the mid 1800's a series of new diagnostic instruments— the stethoscope, the ophthalmoscope, largynscope—began to extend the physician's powers in clinical examination. — A second set of diagnostic technologies—the microscope and x-ray, chemical and bacteriological tests, and machines that generate data on the patient's physiological condition—produced data seeming independent of the physician's judgement."

As mentioned earlier, the introduction of mechanistic science caused dramatic improvements in the physical treatment of patients' problems. The treatment of acute infections, trauma and the correction of hereditary problems (dental abscesses with antibiotics, automobile accidents with the reparative techniques of oral surgery and the correction of malocclusions with orthodontics) are examples of these accomplishments.

Mechanistic science also brought along the attitudes and beliefs of the scientist—one who is an objective observer of phenomena, who believes there is a physical answer to all problems. These attitudes have resulted in the doctor viewing the person who has a disease as an object with a physical problem that needs detached scientific diagnosis and treatment. These attitudes and beliefs knowingly or unknowingly have become wedges between the doctor and patient. They have resulted in comments like, "I'm sure he is a good doctor but, he doesn't seem to care or listen to me." A patient said more bluntly about a surgeon, "He did a good job, but he has the personality of a brick." These objective dispassionate attitudes and beliefs of doctors have resulted in the loss of the feeling, sentient dimensions of respect, compassion, empathy and caring in the doctor-patient relationship.

Western Behavioral Sciences Institute described their search to go beyond the mechanistic approach in this way:

> "We are seeking research methods and a scientific approach that will view man not as a cluster of functions and subsystems, but as an individual—an experiencing, feeling, acting person. In other words, we believe that mechanistic approaches, so successful in the physical sciences, are not entirely adequate for the study of human beings, and need to be supplemented with a more humanistic approach."

"The Good Old Days"

Comments are made about the loss by modern dentists and physicians of the bedside manner that existed in the days before science assumed the dominant role in health care. There is a tendency to idealize the past; to look at the good old days as ideal times. No doubt, the Currier and Ives scenario of the kindly old family dentist or physician caring for his patients is flawed through the mists of memory. Compared to modern dentists and physicians, he was limited in what he could do technically. The environment of his time—the lack of drugs, telephones, technology and treatments we now have—made his humanness the primary skill he had to offer his patients.

He treated the patient in the home, church, barber shop, saloon or work place. Often the treatment was of a first aid type or relied on folk remedies. The dentists and physicians of the 1800's learned their professions through an apprenticeship with older physicians and dentists. They often combined the skills of medicine and dentistry with barbering, farming or other vocations. In contrast to today, he knew his patients within the context of his family, his church, his work and his play. He saw his patient's lifestyle in relation to the patient's everyday environment. He went into the patient's home, workplace, church or community to treat him. He did not see him in his office or a hospital. Paul Starr described this doctor as "a local traveler who knew the interior of his patient's homes and private lives more deeply than others in the community."

Doctors lost their relationship with the human dimensions of patients' lives along their path to more knowledge and technology of the physical dimensions of health care.

For many dentists (and other health care doctors) it is difficult to know if these are the "best of times or the worst of times." When they look at the knowledge and techniques available to treat their patients, it seems to be the best of times. For many dentists it is the worst of times when they look at the loss of the sense of meaning, fulfillment and enrichment they receive from their profession. In losing (or never having) a caring relationship with patients, dentists have lost contact with what gives meaning, fulfillment and enrichment to their professional lives.

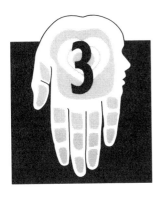

On Caring

The word care is commonly used in dentistry. The term dental care is used generically to describe the various procedures and actions that dentists use in treating their patients. In this context, care means "to watch over, to attend to, to be responsible for, to provide for, to protect." This type of care refers to external actions the dentist provides out of a sense of duty or obligation to do what is best for his patient. It means providing excellence in the dental services he renders to his patients.

These external actions are an integral part of dental care, but as Teilhard de Chardin wrote in *The Phenomenon of Man*, "coextensive to their without, there is a within to things" that "the time has come to realize that an interpretation of the universe—even a positivist one—remains unsatisfying unless it covers the interior as well as the exterior of things: mind as well as matter." The doctor's training, culture and legal requirements have made him a skeptic when he needs to be a hopeful realist in caring for his clients. In developing caring doctor-patient relationships, I am not referring to the without of care, I am referring to the within of care. I am referring to the act of caring for patients or clients. Milton Mayeroff's definition of caring as "helping the other grow" is a good beginning point for clarifying what kind of caring I am referring to. Specifically, a caring doctor-patient relationship is based upon the doctor's intent to help the patient or client to grow and heal because of their relationship with him.

What Caring Means

Mayeroff wrote in his book *On Caring*, "To care for someone, I must know many things. I must know for example who the other is, what his powers and limitations are, what his needs are and what is conducive to his growth; I must know how to respond to his needs, and what my own powers and limitations are." It is this act of caring that heals the chasm between the dentist and his patient. It also is a very tangible part of the client's growth and healing. Several studies have shown that effective doctor-patient relationships increase the patients' compliance with his treatment recommendations (Church, Moretti and Ayer 1980, Gardiner and Sudin, 1976, Garity, 1981). A study by Kaplan and Greenfield, 1989, suggested that better health outcomes and more rapid recovery resulted from more effective doctor-patient relationships. In dentistry, McNeill did a study that used several dentists who used the same treatment and techniques in treating patients with TMD dysfunction. One dentist had statistically better results in treating his patients. Upon investigation, McNeill discovered that the people he was treating felt that he cared more about them and the success of their treatment.

What Caring Asks

Caring asks the dentist to drop his mask of professionalism and to enter the world of the patient. Caring asks the dentist to be fully present, to be authentic and congruent in his interactions with his patients and with himself. Caring asks the dentist to be fully human in his relationships with his patients. The intent to help the patient grow and heal provides the way for the dentist to care. It is this intent that provides the avenue for the dentist to actualize his potential as a healing catalyst and to give meaning and direction to his professional life. Caring dispels the barrenness that inhabits some dentist's professional life. Caring is established through creating healthy relationships with patients. Relationships are the vehicles through which dentists care for their clients. Caring gives the dentist the opportunity to give of himself to his clients through his practice of dentistry.

Caring is communicated through non-judgmental attitudes, words, gestures and affirming touch. This type of caring comes from the heart. The mind follows along to help us understand what this kind of caring means. The doctor uses the caring of his head, hands and heart to help the client heal.

Levels of Caring

I have discovered that there are levels of caring, and through my practice of dentistry my caring broadens and deepens. This path has been the most difficult and the most rewarding thing I have done. If you had asked me early in my dental career if I cared for my patients, I would have looked at you as if you were crazy and answered, "of course I care." If you looked at my interactions with patients, you would have seen that I engaged in a superficial kind of caring. I asked what my patients were doing in their life. I asked about their children, spouses, work and hobbies. I called after their appointment to see how they were doing. I sent birthday cards on their birthday. I did their dental work as well as I could.

Most of these activities were to meet my needs and not the needs of my patients. I hoped by being seen as nice they would accept my recommendations for treatment and refer people to me. It was also a way to fill the time between giving the anesthetic and beginning their dental work. My caring was based on using my relationship with my patients to fulfill my needs. This type of caring did not meet the description of caring described in the previous paragraphs. I thought that care was something I dispensed like prescriptions. Caring was something I did for and to my patient.

It was through time and hard life lessons that I have come to my understanding of the central role that caring plays in my life. When I truly care for my patients, my life feels enriched and fulfilled. It is a quid pro quo phenomenon. The more I give, the more I receive.

An Illustration

The following story is illustrative of the difference this kind of caring makes in my patient's life and in my life. Several years ago, a woman came to see me because she had broken a tooth. She told me that she was extremely phobic about having dental work done. I did an examination and co-diagnosis and helped her understand what dental problems she had and what treatment was needed to correct the problems. She scheduled an appointment for a cleaning. Five minutes into the cleaning she sat up and said, "I can't stay, I need to leave" and she left. Over the next four to five years she would periodically come in with a broken tooth but would only have a cleaning done. During this time we empathized with her fears of dental work and cared for her. She did not have any dental work done.

Then we received a call on a Monday morning. She said: "I have broken a tooth on the upper left side and it hurts. I want to come in and have all my dental work done when possible." We scheduled her that afternoon to fill a cancellation that had occurred. She came in and said, "I have been visualizing since Saturday about having this work done, let's go." She sat in the dental chair and we prepared all of the maxillary posterior teeth for onlays or crowns. She was relaxed and tolerated the preparations, impressions, registrations and temporization well. At the conclusion of the appointment, I asked her what had made the difference in her feelings about having the dental work done. She said, "I now feel safe and cared for here."

We hugged each other in gratitude for the reciprocal roles both of us had played in her dental treatment. She felt good about herself and what she had accomplished, and I felt good about my self and what I had accomplished through caring for her.

Reciprocal Caring

A question is asked, "Is it possible to care in this way without being overwhelmed by the pain, grief, suffering and anxiety that our patients bring with their illnesses." Another question that is asked is: "Won't patients take advantage of you if you care in this way?" Patients will not take advantage of you if you care. They will reciprocate with gratitude and appreciation. Dentists deal with pain and suffering on a daily basis. Our training has taught us to be objective and dispassionate; to keep our humanness hidden in treating our patients pain and suffering. Yet it is our humanness, our caring, our feeling of being needed, of being of help to another, our compassion, humor, joy, pain, suffering, hopes, fears and love that help our patients and ourselves to grow and heal. If we withhold our humanness, we hide the very ingredients that give meaning and direction to our own lives and impair our ability to help our clients grow and heal.

It seems to be a paradox. The qualities that dentists feel should be hidden to protect themselves from their own, and their patients pain and suffering become the qualities that enable them to move through their own pain and suffering. In addition, they help their patient's pain and suffering. Andras Angyal said, "We are restless when we are not needed, because we feel 'unfinished,' "incomplete" and we can only get completed in and through these relationships. We are motivated to search not only for what we lack and need but also for that for which we are needed, what is wanted from us."

Developing or Enhancing a Caring Doctor-Patient Relationship

How do dentists go about developing or enhancing a caring doctor-patient relationship? How do dentists keep a caring relationship from becoming another should do item on an already lengthy list? I feel the answer lies in understanding the dynamics of helping relationships. Fortunately, there is an abundant amount of help to learn how to become effective in creating helping relationships. This help comes from research done in the field of humanistic psychology.

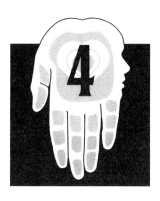

Helping
Relationships

Bob Barkley, a dentist who pioneered humanistic approaches in dentistry, felt that what he did to help a person become healthier was never better than the strength of his relationship with his clients. This belief reflected his feeling of the importance of the doctor-patient relationship in helping his clients heal. If the strength of a doctor-patient relationship is so important to a client's health, healing and ability to learn, what is known about helping relationships? How do helping relationships help dentists become more effective and caring in their relationships with their clients? What research has been done on helping relationships and the doctor-patient relationship? Is there research to support the importance of a caring doctor-patient relationship in the healing of the patient?

In the 1940's, a third force in psychology was emerging through the work of several people. This work became known as perceptual or humanistic psychology. In 1962, Sutich wrote:

> "Humanistic Psychology may be defined as the third main branch of the general fields of psychology (the two already in existence being the behavioral and psychoanalytic) and as such, is primarily concerned with those human capacities and potentialities that have little or no systematic place, either in positivist or behaviorist theory or in classical psychoanalytic theory: e.g., love, creativity, self growth, organism, basic need gratification, self actualization, higher values, being, becoming, spontaneity, play, humor, affection, naturalness, warmth, ego, transcendence, objectivity, autonomy, responsibility, meaning, fair play, transcendental experience, psychological health, and related concepts."

Rogers' Findings

In the 1940's, Carl Rogers started exploring the conditions present in effective counseling relationships. Rogers central hypothesis was: "Individuals have within themselves vast resources for self-understanding and for altering their self-concepts, basic attitudes, and self-directed behavior; these resources can be tapped if a definable climate of facilitative psychological attitudes can be provided."

Rogers' research showed that the presence of three conditions—genuineness or congruence, unconditional positive regard and empathy—in the therapeutic relationship, facilitated a growth promoting climate for clients.

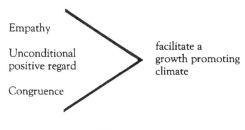

Empathy

Unconditional positive regard

Congruence

facilitate a growth promoting climate

Figure 1.

His research over the years showed that these conditions applied in any relationship where the development of the person was a goal. Examples he gave were relationships between therapist and client, teacher and student, parent and child, doctor and patient, leader and group, manager and employee. Most recently these conditions have been used between adversaries in conflict from the most personal to global.

He described genuineness, realness or congruence in the therapist as "putting up no professional front or personal facade—being the feelings and attitudes that are flowing within at the moment. The term 'transparent' catches the flavor of this condition. — There is a close matching between what is being experienced at the gut level, what is present in awareness, and what is expressed to the client."

He described unconditional positive regard as a nonpossessive "prizing, acceptance, caring or cherishing" of the client. The third condition of empathic understanding meant that "the therapist senses accurately the feelings and personal meanings that the client is experiencing and communicates that understanding to the client. — We think we listen, but we rarely do listen with real understanding, true empathy. Yet listening, of this very special kind, is one of the most potent forces for change that I know."

Rogers felt that this facilitative climate enabled the client to develop more caring attitudes toward themselves, to listen more accurately to their inner experiencing, to become more real and genuine and "to be the true, whole person."

Foundational Tenets of Humanistic Psychology

The following descriptions of the foundational tenets of humanistic psychology draw heavily on the work of Rogers and Arthur Combs, two of the pioneering theorists in perceptual-humanistic psychology.

Humans Are Basically Trustworthy

Rogers said that a human "is a basically trustworthy member of the human species, whose deepest characteristics tend toward development, differentiation, cooperative relationships; whose life tends fundamentally to move from dependence to independence; whose impulses tend naturally to harmonize into a complex and changing pattern of self-regulation; whose total character is such as to tend to preserve and enhance self and species and perhaps to move toward further evolution."

Rogers had a deep abiding faith in the ability of people to make choices that were best for them when a facilitative climate was present. He felt that while a person's behavior could be bad, his nature was not bad.

In health care, this trust is manifested in the belief that clients can be trusted to make health care decisions that are appropriate for them when they are included in the process of making decisions in a facilitative climate.

Formative Tendency

There is a tendency present in the universe toward increased order and complexity on both the organic and inorganic level. The universe is always building, becoming more complex and creating as well as deteriorating. There is a basic drive toward maintenance and enhancement of self in every cell. Helping professions depend upon this basic drive. Persons can, will and must move toward health if the way seems clear. Rogers called this the formative tendency. Szent-Gyorgyi used the term syntropy, and Whyte and Sheldrake called it morphic resonance. This tendency is present in space, microorganisms, in more complex organic life and in human beings. In health care, the person moves toward wholeness, integration and unification, by potentiating their healing systems, whether it is by medication, nutrition, surgery, meditation, imaging or counseling.

Wholeness

Human beings are more than the sum of their parts. They are not just physical beings, emotional beings, intellectual beings, but a complex, integrated whole in which these aspects all contribute to the delightful uniqueness of each person in relation to the world he lives within, much as a wave is part of an ocean. The wave has its distinctive nature, but it is embedded in the whole of the ocean. How a person lives his life influences the whole. When his life is out of balance, his environment is out of balance. The principle of wholeness is utilized in dentistry when all aspects of a person's life (physical, emotional, financial, intellectual, social and spiritual) are considered in developing a treatment plan.

Perceptual World

People behave in terms of how they perceive the world in their own unique ways. They do not behave in terms of objective external criteria. All behavior depends on the person's perceptions—the personal meanings that exist for the individual at the moment of behaving especially the perceptions about self and the world. Our behavior is determined by how we see things from our own frame of reference and not by external objective criteria. To help our clients we need to see things from their viewpoint. We need to walk in their shoes and to lay our frame of reference aside and enter their world nonjudgementally before making conclusions based upon our objective, scientific judgement. Our judgement is a tool to help. It should not be enforced independent of the patient's world view.

Interdependence

The relationship between the professional and client is an inter-dependent one in which the client is viewed as a responsible member of a problem solving, growth creating team. The professional does not manipulate, coerce, badger or bribe toward an end he has chosen. The professional and client both participate in the decision process. The hierarchical relationship between professional and patient is viewed as a hindrance to the healing of the patient. The term patient is abandoned because of its intimation of dependence, of meekness, of subservience to the professional. The term client is used to recognize that in a facilitative climate the person has the resources to solve his problems.

Motivation

According to Combs, motivation springs from personal needs and meanings and not from external manipulation by others. People are motivated—at all times, in all places and under any circum-stances—by the need to enhance the concept they have of them-selves. People do things for their own reasons, not the reasons of others. The goal of helping becomes a positive one of ministering to a trustworthy person. It calls for ways of helping that encourages and facilitates growth by creating conditions of freedom that will enable the person to move toward the degree of fulfillment possible for them at that time. It is a question of aiding, helping, facilitating and assisting rather than coercing, manipulating, cajoling, or brib-ing persons to better things. In dentistry, the client's motivation springs from the personal need to be without pain, to be healthy, to look good, to feel good, to be comfortable, to function well. Dentists do not motivate their clients to action; they create conditions in which the client motivates himself.

Maladaptive, Destructive Tendencies

Arthur Combs stated: "The achievement of a satisfactory degree of fulfillment constitutes psychological health. People who are un-successful or frustrated in their attempts to achieve health and fulfillment become ill or maladjusted. Just as the body's failure to achieve proper growth and fulfillment results in physiological dis-ease, so too, failure of the individual to achieve satisfactory fulfill-ment of self means ill health. Disease is a product of blocks to the physical organism's normal tendency to growth and health. In similar fashion, maladjustment is a consequence of blocks to self fulfillment. Psychological ill health is a matter of falling short, a lack of success in the striving for self realization. The maladjusted are the frustrated ones and the seriousness of their condition is almost directly a function of the degree of deprivation they have suffered."

The work of Carl Rogers, Arthur Combs and other humanistic psychologists has had a powerful impact in my personal and professional life. An explanation of how their work has influenced my professional life may make the work of these people relevant to the practice of dentistry.

As I mentioned in the first chapter, early in my career, I noticed the gap that existed between what I knew and what I communicated to my patients. It seemed I was in the adversarial position of arguing with them to convince them to accept the treatment I had recommended. I also experienced similar frustrations in my relationships with my staff.

The First Dr. Becoming Letter

The following letter explains my growing pains as I struggled with implementing the humanistic approach in my practice. I wrote the letter to Avrom and Deborah King after attending a workshop they presented in 1976, on participative management. The letter was published in their newsletter Nexus in March 1977, as "The Odyssey of Dr. Becoming."

"I thought I'd write to let you know how I've spent the six months since our workshop. But now that I'm ready to do that, I can't really tell you a thing that is meaningful until I discuss the past ten years. (Fourteen years, really when we include dental school—as I think we should). When I graduated from dental school, I was convinced that I did not have what it takes to be a good dentist. I had a severe case of bad hands and bad attitude. For me, dental school was a negative experience.

My next two years were spent in the Army. I enjoyed a pleasant tour while acquiring excellent mechanical experience in various aspects of dentistry. Time and motion was the fad at the time. I remember spending hours working on the refinement of time saving techniques. Somehow that seemed important to me. My interest was related to "production," but I didn't have a clear idea of what I meant by "production" or why it was important. I assumed that with "production" I'd make money. Oh well, we all have to begin somewhere.

My time passed quickly and I came to where I joined in practice with an older dentist and a friend from dental school. After three years the senior dentist retired. I had finally arrived. I was now ready to do great things. No one was standing in my way. As a matter of fact, I had a pretty good year. The next year too. I installed Barkley's five day plaque control program—a magic way to open the pearly gates. But the following year showed no improvement—meaning dollars. I was gaining no greater acceptance from my patients. Then Klein and O'Connor came to town with their two ring circus. I wrote an office manual, designed an ideal day, installed computerized billing. Next year was flat again. No appreciable change. So I put in Nitrous Oxide and went to an ASPD meeting. I learned more about analgesic conscious sedation. Gassed the patients. Controlled them more. Raised my fees 10% and gross went up 10%. So did overhead.

One year later. Just keeping up with inflation. Frustrated with my practice. Maybe with dentistry. What else can I do? (Answer—Nothing) Well the old office was too small, too crowded and too tacky. There was no synergistic effect between my partner and me. I saw the answer. Go on my own and build a new office. I did a careful building cost and practice analysis and discovered I couldn't afford a new office. OK, now I can define the problem. So I'll go look for a solution. After all, by this time I had accumulated the benefits of Barkley, Mittleman, Klein, O'Connor, Kilpatrick, nitrous oxide, Olson, computerized billing, etc. My environment was supersaturated. All I missed was one magic ingredient to make the witch's brew crystallize.

Meanwhile, that famous common denominator of all dental practices, gross overhead, was rising in almost exact proportion to my rising fees. I started to wonder what I'm really worth. Without me knowing the answer, the bank said "yes." In the absence of the magic ingredient, I signed a contract for my new building—The Perfect Dental Office.

Just in time, I heard about Omer Reed and accelerated my practice. My four and a half day practice was cut to four days. Reed talked about motivating the person we call the patient— and Maslow. Well, I've tried everything else, may as well try this. So I read Motivation and Personality.

Learned about the hierarchy of needs. Started to relate to people at their level. Someone told me about the Pankey Institute, and I signed up. I'd have bought anything then because I really had a need to know. The new office was scaring me silly. Learned about the balanced cross. Class one to four patients. Technically best dentistry. Reconstruction. Equilibration. Case planning. Participated in learning instead of lecturing. (Why don't dental schools do that?) It was inspiring, really inspiring. For me it was almost a peak experience. Came back. Changed my practice. Told "my girls" about the fantastic new things we were going to do. Started waxing cases. Diagnosing. Stupid, damn patients still wouldn't listen.

Went to Omer's Napili III. Learned about plantrolling and model-building. Gross per hour. Net per hour. Did a 90 second crown prep in four minutes. Talked about gold, silver. Lots of good ideas from Omer. Accelerated my practice to three days a week.

Back to Pankey. Took C-2. There was a small glimmering in the darkness. I think I was finally beginning to understand how teeth work. (It's a shame they don't help you learn that stuff in dental school. The information would have saved me a lot of time.) Came back. Patients still aren't accepting my recommendations as I want (as I deserve?). I understand how teeth work, but they don't understand me. No time to waste. Back to Reed and Napili IV. Learned how to do case presentations. How to close. Watched myself on closed circuit TV. I sounded like a hick with a monotone. Came back. Tried Omer's closing technique on some patients. They closed—the door on their way out. Maybe I'm not Omer. Maybe I need to develop my own way. What if there isn't a magic ingredient?

My new office isn't too far from completion. If there's a magic ingredient, I need it now. Right now. Construction isn't cheap. No choice. I'm hooked. Back to Pankey and C-3. WOW. Now I feel that I can really do an equilibration. I'm understanding how teeth relate to each other and the tissues and structures around them. **For the first time in ten years of practicing dentistry (believe me when I tell you that I was really practicing because I truly didn't know what to do or how to do it), I am technically a competent dentist. I'm doing dentistry I'd proudly show anyone.**

I came home a million miles high. Patients were accepting more. Not what I feel they should. But more. Don't they realize that I'm now the best damn dentist in town? How do I tell them?

Then I heard about this workshop on participative management. Well, I'm a charter subscriber to Nexus. Omer said I need it and I've got too much invested in Omer to not play the hand. No sense in going halfway with him or you. Might as well attend. The new office is done. It's the most beautiful office ever. Open operatories, Cox equipment, skylights, carpet, cedar walls, designer accessories, rental space, beautiful furnishings, big, spacious, Expensive! Maybe you will have the magic ingredient. I hope so.

The folder said to take my staff, so I will. First time I've ever taken them anywhere. Learned a new way of seeing the world. Learned a new way of seeing my staff. New set of buzz words—participative, non-participative, authoritarian, love, facilitate, Rogers, Toffler, Drucker, trust, assertive, aggressive, self-disclosure. I've heard them before. But really, I hadn't heard a thing. My staff seemed to enjoy this. (By the end of the first day, they truly were people, not just my "girls" anymore.) I was bothered by some of my self discoveries. Well, we'll go back and try warmth, respect and empathy, plus all this participative stuff.

Came back. Carkuffed my patients and staff like crazy. Seemed forced. But patient's were responding. And the staff has never been higher. (Are these related?) It's getting easier. Maybe there is something to this. Better find out fast. Have to do some reading.

Started with Carl Rogers' Freedom to Learn. *The first chapters were a little tedious for me, but the last part is dynamite.* **He is saying what I feel, what I've felt.** *It came together in my head as I was reading Rogers. All of it. It's an upside-down, inside-out, boogieing, bumping, mind-blowing peak experience complete with tingles, tears, lumps, perception and expansion of reality. I kept on reading such books as* On Becoming a Person, The Skilled Helper, Art of Helping *and* Helping Relationships.

I was turned on. The workshop experience became whole. Then real. Then vivid. What had happened to me since our being together six months ago is, for me, a miracle. **For the first time in ten years, I am not only competent as a dentist, I am enjoying dentistry. until now, I had overlooked the value of people and the sheer joy of relating to them. Now I get up and I'm eager to go to the people place called a dental office. Now my beautiful office is ever so much more beautiful because it's filled with beautiful people.**

Material rewards are coming. I have good months and not so good months. But I have confidence and acceptance (me of me, me of them, them of me). It will take some time. I've run a lot of people out of here. I'll certainly stumble. Probably fall. But I'll get up **and now I'll learn, grow, prosper from the experiences.** *Along the way, I'll enjoy, doubt, agonize, soar, have fun and respond to challenge.*

Well, I've run out of paper. The tablet is empty, but I am not. It's unfair to have a story without an ending. But how can feelings end? For the first time in my life, I'm becoming, not being. For the first time in my life, I love and accept me. For the first time in my life, I love and accept those whom I work with and those whom we serve."

Sincerely,

Lynn

In Retrospect

It had been a while since I last read this letter. Rereading it brings back the joys and frustrations I experienced because of my journey. There was a frantic search for the magic ingredient to make my practice life fulfilling. I was searching outside myself for the magic solution. There was a persistence in my search. As I struggled, I blamed others for my shortcomings, especially the senior dentist and my dental school friend. As long as I continued to look outside, success eluded me. When I looked inside, I found the path to fulfillment.

Some Learnings

Obviously this period of the middle 1970's was a time of intense learning for me. This learning continues. Some additional learning is:

✦ I realize when I view my patients as equals—when I respect their fears, questions, their right to control their health, their responsibility for their own health and their humanness—I view them as collaborators or partners on a journey we are taking together. I am a companion, a mentor, an educator, a facilitator and guide instead of an authoritarian or benevolent dictator who directs and controls their life. We create an interdependent relationship.

✦ When I enter my clients' world non-judgmentally and try to capture the world from their perspective, my client can express himself more clearly and fully, and I am more able to help him. When I understand what is going on in his life, I can tailor my treatment for him and his situation. I do not mechanically recommend treatment that does not fit into the context of his life. An example is: if a client is going through a stressful divorce or job change, I do not start invasive, elective dental treatment. I discuss with the client his choices and facilitate his decision making on having dental work done in relation to the other events occurring in his life. When I am unable to do this, the outcome clinically and behaviorally is less than I hoped.

✦ People do things for their reasons and not mine. My training and experience as a dentist gives me a particular world view. What I value and the choices I make are often different from the choices my client would make. The rightness of my knowledge as a dentist is not enough to motivate them, unless it has personal meaning for them. My challenge is to help my clients recognize and value needs and wants they did not know they had. Dental disease is often insidious; the client is not aware they have dental decay, gum disease or malocclusion until it hurts. Without swelling, bleeding or pain they may not feel that the dental work is a priority in their life. They would rather buy a new car, carpet the house, take a trip or buy clothes instead of having the dental work done.

✦ I am more effective with people I like, who have had experiences similar to my experiences and hold values similar to my values. If my clients have had similar experiences, I can use analogies or experiences from my own life to help them understand the need for the dental treatment. Also, I can't help everyone that comes to see me. Sometimes, the client and I are not a good match.

✦ My clients have been my greatest educators. My experiences with my clients have given me most of my opportunities for learning. These opportunities have been both rewarding and frustrating. I have come to trust that uneasiness, discomfort, joy and excitement are all signs that an opportunity to learn and grow is present. If I use these as grist for my mill, positive change will occur. My client's feedback, criticism, suggestions, lack of responsiveness, support and compliments have all been stimuli for change. My experience and wisdom have broadened because of these interactions with my clients. These interactions have helped me become less provincial and able to relate to more people.

✦ People have different strengths, weaknesses, beliefs, values and behavior than I have. They are not wrong because their beliefs and values are different from mine. If I can understand these beliefs and values, then I appreciate the differences and learn from them. I did not discover this obvious fact until I was in my middle 30's. Before that time, I naively assumed I was right and anyone who differed with me was wrong.

✦ If I communicate in a way that is not congruent with what I am feeling, then the communication is not as effective or deep. The client experiences dissonance and they don't trust what I say. A few years ago, I attended a course on dental implants. I returned to my office with a born again fervor to do an implant. I recommended one to the first likely candidate. I have not seen him since.

✦ The more open I am to trusting my client's knowledge of himself, the better the clinical result will be. I have talked clients into having a procedure done when they did not feel it should be done. I used my power and authority as a doctor to persuade them to have the treatment done. In retrospect, I did the treatment because of my needs and not those of my client.

✦ How a person feels emotionally influences the person's physical health and disease. There have been times when I corrected the physical aspect that seemed to have caused the problem only to have the problem continue or worsen. When this happens, there is usually an underlying emotional problem that is unresolved. The physical pain does not stop until the emotional problem is resolved. I work with people who have chronic pain related to occlusal/muscle and temporomandibular joint dysfunction. I have done everything physically possible to correct the problem (splint therapy, biofeedback, physical therapy, occlusal equilibration, diet change and acupuncture) only to be frustrated by the intractability of the problem. The pain disappeared when the person left their spouse, changed jobs, graduated or entered psychotherapy.

The opposite is also true. Physical problems lead to emotional problems. There can be multiple causes of disease that include the physical, emotional and spiritual.

✦ Fear is a significant deterrent to communication. Coming to a health care professional may provoke anxiety and create barriers to effective communication. This fear and anxiety can be overtly or covertly expressed as hostility toward the dentist. This hostility occurs because the dentist is physically and emotionally entering an intimate and very sensitive area. This fear and hostility may, despite the doctor's effectiveness as a communicator, be enough to create barriers to effective communication. The recognition of this fact, has the potential to relieve the dentist's frustration at his inability to communicate with his clients. Information given in the presence of fear and anxiety is often not received or is incompletely understood. Often, other people on the dental team can communicate more effectively with patients than the doctor. They do not carry the emotional baggage that the doctor does as the authority or as "the doctor."

✦ I enjoy being listened to and deeply appreciate when a client recognizes my feelings, expresses gratitude for what I have done for him or gives me a hug. I am connected with my clients through my relationship with them. I am influenced by them and may feel what they feel. If I feel as if I have given to them without a return then I feel drained, stressed or burnt out. Dentistry can be lonely work without understanding and compassion from clients, family, co-workers and colleagues. When I don't have this understanding, I am like a plant without food and water; I wither, become limp, even lifeless. When I experience reciprocal relationships with clients, co-workers or colleagues, I blossom.

✦ The client has power and control over his own health, disease and illness. He is responsible for his health and healing. No one else can do this; the client is the only one who can respond to the events and conditions that led to his health or disease. The client is the one in which the healing occurs. The doctor does not have the sovereign right to diagnose and treat without the client's active involvement. The client heals himself. The doctor is an adjuvant—a healing catalyst—who helps or facilitates the client's healing by his presence, knowledge, caring, treatment, counseling and recommendations.

Keystones to Health and Healing

Effective, caring doctor-patient relationships are keystones to the health, wellness and healing of the client and the health and wellness of the dentist. Humanistic psychology through its research on effective helping relationships points the way for dentists to learn how to become more adept in their relationships with their clients. My own experience in developing these relationships has deepened and expanded my understanding of the dynamics of the doctor-patient relationship. What are the characteristics that differentiate the caring doctor-patient relationship from the traditional relationship between doctor and patient?

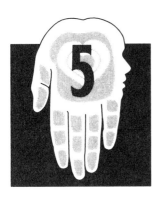

Doctor-Patient Relationships

What are the characteristics that differentiate the caring doctor-patient relationship from the traditional relationship between doctor and patient? A relationship begins anytime a doctor and patient have an interaction. It may be of short duration or a long standing one. It may be a facilitative relationship, a destructive relationship or a neutral relationship. What is a relationship? Usually a relationship is defined as: "the quality or state of being related; connection." Some synonyms for relationship are: tie, association, affinity, likeness, link, kinship, rapport, interaction. These are beginning points for defining a doctor-patient relationship.

A comparison of the traditional doctor-patient relationship and a facilitative relationship will clarify the distinctions between the two relationships.

Characteristics of a Traditional Doctor-Patient Relationship

In the traditional relationship, the doctor is viewed as an all knowing authority figure whose responsibility is to cure the disease or repair the injury. The patient is a passive, dependent, recipient of the doctor's ministrations. The patient unquestioningly complies with the doctor's instructions. The doctor is viewed as perfect, one who does not make mistakes. The patient does not take too much of the doctor's time, because the doctor's time is more important that the patient's. The doctor's focus is on efficiency. The doctor is not concerned with the patient's feelings and concerns. He focuses on the prevention and elimination of the disease or the symptoms.

In the traditional relationship, symptoms, pain and disease are wholly negative and the doctor focuses on their elimination. He relies solely on quantitative data (tests, ranges, cultures) to make his decisions regarding care. The patient is not responsible for the conditions that have led to his disease, because illness and disease only come from without because of bacteria, accidents, and trauma. The doctor is the healer and the patient is the recipient of his healing. Therefore, the doctor is the one that is responsible for the cure and if the cure does not work, the doctor or the health care system is at fault.

Characteristics of the Person-Centered Relationship

The person-centered or facilitative doctor-patient relationship is one in which there is an attitude of service present in the doctor. The patient is a collaborator or partner in the relationship (because the word patient implies a dependent relationship with the doctor, the word client is used in describing the person who comes to the doctor for care). The doctor understands his primary role is to use his technical excellence and the intangible qualities of his humanness—caring, compassion, vulnerability, genuineness, wholeness, respect, valuing and empathy—to help his client heal.

The client is responsible for his health and illness. In this definition, responsible means the client has the ability to respond to his illness, trauma or disease. The client is not a passive recipient of illness or disease but a person who has within himself the necessary resources to facilitate his healing. The doctor is recognized as human and part of his humanness is his potential to make mistakes, not from negligence or incompetence, but from his humanness. The doctor's caring is a vital part of the client's healing. The context of the client's life—his attitudes, beliefs, values, feelings, lifestyle, relationships—contributes to his health or disease.

Pain and disease can give information about disharmony in the client's life. This disharmony may be a result of his attitudes, beliefs, values, feelings, lifestyle and relationships. The doctor includes subjective criteria, such as the patients feelings, concerns and ideas and the doctor's own intuition, feelings and ideas in his evaluation of the problem. The doctor is concerned with helping the client achieve or return to a feeling of well being and not just the elimination of the disease or symptoms.

Person-centered or facilitative approaches do not abandon the strengths of the traditional doctor-patient relationship, but build, integrate and expand upon it. There is a difference in attitudes, beliefs and values between the traditional and facilitative doctor-patient relationships.

The Importance of Values and Beliefs

Combs sheds some light on his intriguing question "What Makes a Good Helper?" Since the 1960's, Combs and his colleagues have done a series of research projects to explore the question of what differentiates a good helper from a poor one. They have studied counselors, teachers, nurses, supervisors, Episcopal priests, professors and public officials. (I have done a survey to study this question with dentists and have had similar preliminary results to Comb's research.)

Their research found that it was not the methods or the knowledge of the helper that was important, but the difference was in the belief systems of the helpers. Clear differences emerged in the research studies between good and poor helpers' perceptual organizations or belief systems. To date, they have found five major areas of helper belief systems that relate to effective practice. To help the reader adapt Comb's research to dentistry, I have applied their work to a facilitative doctor-patient relationship.

Area 1. Sensitivity, Empathy

The doctor is sensitive to and concerned with how things seem to the client with whom he interacts. He uses this as a basis for his own behavior in responding to the client. He is concerned with the perceptions of the client, as well as their overt behavior. He sees himself in relation to people instead of things; he is more concerned with the client as a vital human being, instead of a problem to be cured or solved. Ineffective doctors are more concerned with how things seem to themselves.

Area 2. Beliefs about People

Effective doctors typically possess positive views about people. They see them as able, dependable, worthy, friendly and helpful. The doctor perceives his clients as having the capacities to deal with their problems. Clients have within themselves the resources to promote their own healing. The doctor regards his clients as trustworthy instead of untrustworthy. The doctor trusts his client's knowledge and ability to make decisions regarding their health. Ineffective doctors approach people with suspicion, doubt and apathy.

Area 3. Feelings about Self

Effective doctors see themselves as enough—as liked, wanted, accepted, able people of dignity and integrity. They see themselves identifying with people instead of apart from them. They see themselves as part of the whole of humankind and not as isolated from others. They enjoy working with people and are drawn toward people. The doctor has a positive view of himself as having the resources to deal with his problems and the problems of others. When a problem arises, the doctor feels challenged instead of intimidated and feels in control of his environment.

Ineffective doctors see themselves as unliked, unwanted, unacceptable and have doubts about their abilities.

Area 4. Purposes

Effective doctors' purposes tend to be freeing. The doctor's role is to serve as a facilitator to help the client become healthier, instead of controlling or manipulating the client to choose the means and ends the doctor has chosen. They behave altruistically instead of narcissistically. The doctor is motivated by a concern for the patient's well being in addition to the treatment outcome. They trust that by providing altruistic care their own needs will be met. They display a trust that in giving of themselves they will also receive.

Effective doctors are concerned with larger instead of smaller meanings. The doctor sees himself in terms of a larger perspective and larger whole. This relationship to a larger whole gives meaning and direction to their personal and professional life. There is a sense of mission and purpose to their profession. This mission and purpose gives a meaningful vision to their practice.

Area 5. Authenticity and Methods

The authenticity of whatever the helper does in the relationship is the most important factor in being a good helper. Combs' and associate's research has shown that authenticity is more important than the methods employed. Effective doctors are self-revealing. Their sincerity, honesty and clarity of purpose are communicated no matter what method they use. Ineffective doctors tend to be self-concealing. They are their roles, their purposes and hold themselves aloof from their clients.

The effective doctor is self-revealing instead of self-concealing. The doctor feels comfortable in revealing his thoughts and feelings to the client and does not fear the clients' response. The doctor is genuine and congruent in the expression of these thoughts and feelings. They feel the expression of thoughts and feelings is significant and important.

Combs believed that to be of help, to help another grow and heal, the helper needs a set of clarified personal values and beliefs that have personal meaning for him and that they have a tested systematic theory. Life experience, training in his field, a trust in people, the intent to help and goals to seek are also important. These beliefs and values enable the doctor to enjoy his profession, to feel a calling and to look forward to helping his clients.

I hope these values and beliefs are not viewed as additional demands in an already stressful profession. I simply believe that when they are present, doctors' lives function better. There is more joy in the practice of dentistry and in relationships with clients and colleagues. When they exist there is an enhanced opportunity for the client to heal. When these values and beliefs are present, doctors transcend the usual constraints that their traditional beliefs and values about being scientific and professional impose upon their personal and professional lives.

These facilitative beliefs are not present for me every moment of every day. I still have moments of doubt, frustration, fear, of wondering if I chose the right profession—if there is an easier way of earning a living. There are still people who drain my energy. However, when I have the intent to help my clients grow and heal, my experience of the joy of caring expands, and my moments of doubt, frustration and fear diminish.

Becoming Adept at Caring Doctor-Patient Relationships

How do doctors become adept at caring doctor-patient relationships? There are several characteristics of effective helping relationships. They include: empathy, authenticity, congruence, positive beliefs about others and self and a global holistic perspective.

How does a doctor create these characteristics if he feels he doesn't have them? These characteristics exist while living, from seeking to grow, from having the intent to be a good person, an authentic, fully functioning person. It is a process of letting what is inherent blossom, much as a seed becomes a beautiful flower, of supplying nurturing conditions to actualize our inherent potential. Does this sound too abstract? I will be more specific by relating how I learned to help my clients.

◆ *Reading, writing and studying.* I love reading and have used reading for acquiring knowledge about helping relationships. This knowledge is not a veneer, but through the years it has seeped into the core of my being and has become a part of me. Reading meaningful books has struck a deep chord in me. It seems that when I am in need of support or guidance, a book will come into my life that answers the questions I am asking at the time. I have been like the bottom of an hour glass that has been filled by books with knowledge and understanding.

Writing is a way for me to reach within and allow what is inside to flow out and to record this on paper. The act of writing provides an experience of discipline to make clear and specific what is often a vague concept or feeling. Writing enables me to turn the hour glass over and give back what I have learned. I have written in personal journals, newsletters, professional journals, magazines and in books.

Study is a means of massaging, kneading, playing and giving meanings to the learning I receive from reading and writing.

◆ *Reflecting, meditating, contemplating.* There are times when I feel a need to be quiet, to reflect, to listen. I am learning to trust the wisdom that is available to me through these ways of being. When I can still my mind from chattering, this wisdom flows from a deep place. I use deep breathing, meditative music, walks in the woods and by the lake near my home, hiking in the mountains, sitting by a stream, bicycle rides and skiing to help me quiet my mind and open to this wisdom.

◆ *Workshops.* Workshops, particularly person-centered workshops, have been the most effective way of accelerating my learning. I have felt quicker, more profound change and growth in these workshops than in any other ways of learning.

The environment of a person-centered workshop seems to fit and help me change. The opportunity to risk new behavior in a supportive, caring environment has been most helpful to me in my learning and growth.

✦ *Mistakes.* I am a stubborn person. My way of learning from my mistakes is to hit an obstacle head first, back up, gear down and run harder into the same obstacle, then back up and run harder with my knees higher and my head lower into the same obstacle. Over time, I have learned this is not the most effective way of learning. I have reduced (but not eliminated) the number of times I run into an obstacle before I stop and look around to see if there is a better way of solving the problem. Now, I usually walk around the obstacle to see if I can gain a different perspective to solve the problem.

Some of my most significant learnings have occurred from my mistakes. My mistakes always offer me an opportunity to learn. The root meaning of sin is a term from archery that means "off the mark." They show me when I am off the mark and allow me opportunities to correct. Henry Tanner believes a great educational event occurs when you recognize a mistake the second time you make it.

✦ *Family, clients, colleagues.* What better people to help you with relationships than those closest to you. Paradoxically, my behavior in my close relationships was the hardest to change. This change occurred later, it was like a law of physics—the closer someone or something is to you, the harder it is to change. The constant, often frustrating feedback from these close relationships has provided me with the most opportunities to learn and grow.

I am deeply moved when I receive validation from those closest to me that I am making progress; that I was practicing what I preached. I feel good when I see the people in my life responding with empathy, respect, gratitude and caring because I know that my interaction with those closest to me provides a valid mirror of where I am in my life.

✦ *Mentors.* I have been blessed with many mentors in my life. They have been people who have shared their wisdom, caring and guidance to me on my journey through life. They have been my guides, counselors, wise men and women, and friends. They have been down the path I am traveling and have provided help, insight, understanding, knowledge and compassion as I make my journey. Through my association with them I have found knowledge, wisdom and understanding of myself and my journey. Practically, they have helped me avoid many obstacles and lessen my times of feeling lost and frustrated.

✦ *Time.* Becoming adept at caring doctor-patient relationships is developmental and takes time. Changing attitudes, beliefs and habits is not subject to quick fixes and short cuts. Patience is necessary or needs to be learned to make fundamental change.

The process of learning, growth and change is not a linear one—directional process. It involves risk, failure, success, falling down and getting up again, of "keeping on keeping on." In my experience the rewards are worth the price I have paid. Because of my journey, I have gained greater compassion and understanding of myself and my clients from the experiential process of learning. The process of discovery and learning begins with the first step. The first step is a unique one for you. It is a matter of trusting the process of learning and then making a leap of faith.

Our experience of our own learning will help us when we help our clients learn new behavior or new understandings of their health. We need to be teachers or facilitators of learning to help clients understand their health problem.

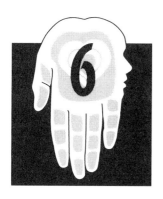

Learning
About Learning

These are challenging times for dentists. Various research papers have suggested that 60–80% of illnesses are lifestyle related. In dentistry, these figures are higher as the research on the causes of dental caries and periodontal disease shows. Temporomandibular joint dysfunction, oral and dental trauma are other examples of lifestyle related diseases in dentistry. Heart disease, cancer, ulcers, back problems, accidents, child abuse and substance abuse are other common lifestyle related diseases.

Dental disease is intimately related to the health of the rest of the body. The prevention or elimination of dental disease contributes to the health of the whole body. The following quotes emphasize this relationship. Charles C. Bass, M.D. in the May 1965 issue of the American Heart Journal wrote, "In almost all ailments of the heart caused by bacteria, the source of infection is known to be the pathologic and infected environment of the teeth. . . . the health, welfare and even life itself, of persons who have heart conditions which predispose to infection may depend on prevention and control of dental disease." Louis H. Mayo M.D. said, "Preventive dentistry can extend human life ten years." Sir William Osler mentioned, "There is not one single thing in preventive medicine as important as oral hygiene and the preservation of the teeth."

Dentists spend most of their time treating oral and dental disease and trauma with surgery, various types of prosthesis, restorative and orthodontic techniques. They treat their client's oral and dental disease with mechanistic and pharmaceutical approaches. If a client has dental decay, the decay is removed and restored with a dental material. If a client has periodontal disease, the disease is treated with scaling and planing or surgery. Why do dentists need to understand how people learn if most of their time is spent doing mechanical procedures for their clients? This question is often asked in relation to why dentists should learn more about learning.

Some Rhetorical Questions

The following rhetorical questions come to mind in response to the above question.

1. In order for the dentist to do the crown, the client needs to consent to have the treatment done. How does the dentist help the client accept the need for the crown?
2. Mechanical dental procedures are not done in a vacuum. The dentist needs the clients' active involvement for the procedure to be successful. Even if the dentist does a technically perfect crown, its ultimate success is decided by the client's active involvement in maintaining good oral hygiene and diet and to manage the stress in their lives. Once the crown is cemented and the client walks out the door, the success of the crown depends upon the client. What does the dentist need to know to insure the success of the crown if this success is dependent upon the client's lifestyle?
3. What causes the disease in the first place? What were the factors or conditions that led to the disease? How does the dentist help the client prevent the disease from recurring?
4. If dental caries and periodontal disease are controllable or preventable by lifestyle changes, then what does the dentist need to know to help the client make positive lifestyle changes and practice good oral hygiene?
5. If stress is a major contributor to physical disease, such as myofascial pain dysfunction and periodontal disease, then what does the dentist need to know to help their client manage their stress?
6. If 60–80% of illnesses are lifestyle related, then what skills does the dentist need to enable their patients to change their destructive lifestyle habits?
7. If, as the research in mind/body relationships in disease, proves there is a direct link between the mind, body and emotions, then what does the dentist need to know to help their clients understand how the mind and emotions can heal or create the disease?

Answers to the Rhetorical Questions

The answer to these rhetorical questions is: dentists can be far more effective in helping their clients solve their problems if they learn more about learning. Today, disease patterns are shifting from an acute to a chronic nature of disease. Fries and Crapo stated in

Vitality and Aging: "Years of useful life lost through early death caused by the (historical) acute or infectious diseases have dropped 99.5% in North America over the past 100 years." The chronic, lifestyle illnesses mentioned earlier in this chapter, have become the leading inhibitors of the quality and quantity of life today. A Harvard study showed that hospitals and physicians are not proving effective in preventing or eliminating chronic diseases. A result of this shift is that dentists are confronted with a new environment that requires enhanced skills in their role as counselor and teacher.

Wilson Southam believes that the central issues for modern health care are those of lifestyle and the limiting of self-imposed risks. Research published in the November 10, 1993 issue of the Journal of the American Medical Association, found that nearly one-half of the 2.148 million deaths in 1990 could have been prevented through behavioral changes such as: stopping smoking, eating healthier food, exercising more, shunning alcohol and practicing safe sex. Southam believes that dentistry, through the work done by the people I mentioned in the first chapter, is leading the way to a better model of nonurgency, primary health care. He lists five reasons for his belief.

1. *Self-imposed risks and lifestyle diseases.* To improve people's dental health means changing people's behavior. Dentistry is already in the behavior change and lifestyle disease business because of the lifestyle related nature of dental disease.
2. *The near universality and significance of periodontitis.* Periodontal disease is more of a threat to a person's general health than the public or physicians recognize. The self-care disciplines to control or prevent periodontal disease are the same disciplines essential to preventing or eliminating chronic disease.
3. *The role of the hygienist (dental team) in long range care.* The nature of dental disease and the need for regular visits to a dental office for oral prophylaxis creates ongoing relationships with the dental team. These relationships enable the dental team to become facilitators of change in destructive lifestyle behavior.
4. *The significance of the nonfatal nature of dental disease.* The lack of the threat of death and time pressure, along with the generally healthier condition of dental clients, enables the dental team to build effective helping relationships. This lack enables the dental team to help clients learn health planning and self care skills that apply to their general health and well being.

5. *The impact of the end of dentistry's period of natural monopoly.* Because of the decline in dental disease, the increase in the dentist-client ratio and increased productivity, dentists have strong economic incentives to look for ethical ways to differentiate themselves from competitors. A dental practice based upon processes developed in the behavioral sciences offers a way for dental practices to differentiate themselves.

Dentists Are in the Behavior Change and Lifestyle Business

Dentists have some clients come to see them for help with physical ailments that have their origin in a dysfunctional family, substance abuse, stressful work situations, poor dietary habits, low self-esteem, marital problems, poor physical condition and spiritual barrenness. Dentists need to learn that besides treating and preventing dental disease, they are in the behavior change and lifestyle business. The challenge is to become a teacher and counselor to help clients solve their problems of living. Another challenge is to help them move on to a feeling of well being, integration and wholeness.

A woman in her forties came to see me for a second opinion. She was told by another dentist that she needed an immediate denture and several crowns and bridges on her lower teeth. She was referred to us by a friend to see if there was something else that could be done for her. My examination showed that she had Code 3 and 4 periodontal disease with pockets up to 7–9 millimeters. There were missing teeth on the upper and lower arches. I told her that what the other dentist had told her was a valid recommendation. I asked her how she felt about losing her teeth. She said she dreaded the thought of wearing a denture and was concerned about the cost of the dental treatment.

I asked her about her lifestyle. Did she smoke? Did she eat breakfast? How much stress did she have in her life? She said that she smoked and did not eat breakfast. She thought the stress in her life was low. I told her that in my experience people who smoked and did not eat breakfast had a difficult time controlling periodontal disease. I said if she wanted to try to save her teeth, she would need to stop smoking and improve her diet. I asked her to take some time to think about whether she would be willing to stop smoking and to change her diet. She said she would. One week later, she made an appointment for an Initial Interview and co-diagnosis appointment. She had not smoked for a week and had started eating breakfast. She said she had been extremely stressed from not smoking and had discovered that she had covered her stress by smoking. She said she was willing to do whatever it took to try to save her teeth.

I had served her as a lifestyle counselor and had talked about the necessity of changing the destructive lifestyle habits that were contributing to her periodontal disease. I had become a teacher and counselor to her.

The Meaning of Being a Teacher

As I mentioned in the previous chapters, the beliefs dentists hold are crucial to their effectiveness in helping their clients learn. Most dentists have abandoned their belief in their role as a teacher. Paradoxically, as information, knowledge, technology, drugs and techniques have proliferated, dentists metaphysical link with their role as teachers and counselors has withered. The emphasis in dentistry on efficiency and productivity, the elimination of disease, on making the correct diagnosis, on managing clients, on being scientific and on being professional, led to distancing dentists from their origin as learned men or women, counselors and teachers.

In seeking the etymon, the true sense of a word, the early people sensed a metaphysical link between the meaning of the word and the person, thing or activity it described. The following are derivatives for doctor: Middle English—doctor: teacher, learned man: Old French or Latin—doctor, teacher . of docere, to teach: IndoEuropean—base * dek—to receive, to do what is suitable. An understanding of what it means for a dentist to be a teacher is important, if dentists are to respond to the challenge of being more effective in helping their clients learn how to prevent or manage their problems. I want to be clear about what the word teacher means to me. Dentists have knowledge that can help people become well. A key function of a dentist is to share his knowledge and information with the people he serves. This function fulfills Webster's definition of teaching: to instruct, to give lessons to, but this is an incomplete definition of teaching.

These types of teaching do not necessarily lead to learning. This definition implies that a person is an empty vessel that needs filling. The expression "the mug and jug approach" describes this style of learning. This definition implies that teaching is a one-directional process with the knowledge or instructions descending from teacher to student. The assumption has been that when there is instructing, showing, telling and directing, learning automatically occurs.

Research has shown that this is not true. Human beings have an inherent, natural, trustworthy, incessant desire to learn. This desire to learn is actuated by a search for personal meaning, for the need to know and by a basic drive toward health and wellness. Because of these beliefs, I prefer to broaden the word teacher to include the term facilitator—one who makes learning, growth, change and healing easier. A facilitator makes the person's inherent drive to learn, easier for them to actualize.

What Research Has Shown

What are some research based principles that can help dentists facilitate their client's learning? Again Arthur Combs provides a way for us to understand how to help people learn. The following draws heavily from his book, *A Personal Approach to Teaching: Beliefs That Make A Difference* and my conversations with him.

Combs along with Donald Snygg began developing a theory of persons, which they called a perceptual approach to human behavior, in 1949. "A perceptual view of learning, . . . seeks to produce some change in the behavior of the learner." Behavior in their definition is "only a symptom of what is going on in the learner's perceptual field." Personal meanings or perceptions are regarded as the determinates of behavior.

Learning in Combs' frame of reference, is regarded as the discovery of personal meaning. Any information or experience will affect a person's behavior only to the degree to which the person has discovered the personal meaning for him or her. For example, I had a client who told me she had Huntington's Disease. I had a dim memory from my class in pathology that it was a disease of the nervous system. That memory was about twenty-five years old, and I did not remember much more than I have related. I listened to her as she related what the disease was, how it affected her family and her concerns about how it affected her dentally (she did not have the motivation and manual dexterity to brush and take care of her oral hygiene). We had not seen her for two years, and during that time, she had rapid degenerative breakdown of the periodontal ligament and bone around one of her molars.

Through my research on Huntington's Disease and my experience with her, I now know much more about the disease and it's physical and emotional consequences for my client and her dental health. The personal meaning her disease had to her, and to me as her dentist, lead me to learn about the history, etiology, prognosis and care of Huntington's disease. I also learned how it affected her and her family emotionally.

Perceptual Approaches to Learning

In perceptual terms, learning occurs from the person's discovery of personal meaning. This approach is also called experiential learning. Some basic principles of perceptual/experiential learning are:

+ *Learning is a deeply personal process.* Effective learning includes much more than the acquisition of information or knowledge. It is a deeply personal process that is affected by a person's feelings, emotions, attitudes, self concept and values. Effective learning occurs because of its feeling of personal meaning. This feeling of personal meaning creates emotions that vary from excitement to fear. The feeling of fear or excitement stirs up, puts in motion, calls forth, arouses and increases a response to a learning situation.

Do you remember when you were excited about something—a new technique, a new way of seeing things—and the joy you felt as you pursued learning more about the subject? Conversely, do you remember the fear you felt when you took the National, Regional or State boards and the amount of time you spent in preparation for these examinations?

Some of the most important learning any of us ever has, has nothing to do with more experience or information. Instead, they are dependent upon the deeper and deeper discovery of the meaning of something already known. Combs uses the example of the brotherhood of man. Few of us need more information. Rather we need to discover the deeper meaning of what we already know.

+ *Learning is motivated by personal need.* All behavior is motivated by the basic need of the organism for fulfillment. This includes the process of learning. People do what seems important to them. They ignore or respond with apathy or indifference to what they view as unimportant. Barkley said dentists often give patients solutions to needs they did not know they had. A typical example in dentistry is the presentation of a treatment plan for an equilibration and full or partial reconstruction of the mouth when the client thought they had come in for a cleaning or at the most a few fillings. The client has no way of knowing how this treatment relates to his health, fulfillment or well being, because he was unaware of a problem. Since all information must be related to personal need, learning must be directed at either: the client's existing need or the dentist faces a challenge to help the client discover needs he never knew he had. The hallmark of an effective teacher or dentist is helping students or clients become aware of needs they did not know they had.

✦ *Learning is critically affected by the learner's concept of self.* People learn when they see themselves as capable of learning. When the self concept includes the perception that they are able to learn, then people will learn more easily. English was my weakest subject in college. I received A's and B's in all my subjects except English. I avoided writing and felt inadequate when I needed to write letters to colleagues, friends and clients. I worried about the grammar, conciseness, clarity and syntax. Then I had an article (The Odyssey of Dr. Becoming) published and I received positive feedback from my fellow dentists who said "You write what I feel— Thanks!" This positive response gave me the courage to write more articles. My self concept as a writer changed and I wanted to learn more about the craft of writing. This change in self-concept led to the writing of this book.

✦ *The learner's concept of challenge or threat decides the degree of involvement and learning that takes place.* Effective learning requires getting involved. This involvement is primarily decided by the person's perception of the challenge or threat the learning opportunity presents. The Chinese ideogram for crisis symbolizes both danger and opportunity. People feel challenged when something interests them, and they feel they can handle it successfully. People are threatened when they are confronted by a situation they feel unable to handle.

In dentistry, this is a primary issue dentist's face as they inform their clients about a serious problem. When people feel a threat, they avoid the threatening situation from a fear of and a desire to avoid the perceived consequences. This fear is a result of the meaning to self of the threat. This threat results in two things happening; one is tunnel vision, and the other is defense of existing beliefs.

Relating a diagnosis of a disease that is dreaded by the person can initiate a mist of fear that creates blocks to the client hearing anything the dentist says. Dentists often aggravate this problem by trying to eliminate the block with more information, solutions and explanations. Often, it is better to support the person with empathy, caring and respect instead of delivering more information or explanations.

Informing a client that they have advanced periodontal disease, when they were unaware or when they have dreaded hearing they have it, is an excellent example. Frequently these clients will cancel their appointments or will not do the self care that is necessary to control the disease. Others will attempt to blame the dentist for their periodontal problem. The feeling of threat to self has blocked their ability to respond to the disease through understanding and self care. Options in this circumstance are: responding to their feelings with active listening, providing support through understanding and caring, giving them written material or video tapes or having people talk to them who have successfully controlled periodontal disease. Another option is to have them return in a few days with a close friend or family member to hear what you have to say.

The issue of challenge and threat is a critical one in dentistry. We have had little experience in dental school or post graduate education to help us wind our way through this delicate area. Challenge and threat are perceptual experiences. What challenges and excites one person to learn and grow, will immobilize another. What initially is a threat may later become a life transforming challenge. There is a rich body of writings about people who were diagnosed as having a terminal illness. These people used these life threatening diseases as the stimulus to make changes in their life and survive the illness or disease.

✦ *Learning is deeply influenced by the learner's feeling of belonging or identification.* People learn best when they feel cared for, respected, prized, accepted and feel a sense of belonging. I have learned more from my life experiences when these conditions were present. These conditions enabled me to risk, fail, change, learn and grow. All of my most important learning experiences had these conditions present.

✦ *Meaningful feedback of knowledge or results is essential for effective learning to occur.* Feedback that is maximally useful fulfills the following characteristics.

1. *It is immediate as possible.* The closer the feedback is to the event, the more learning will occur. Most often people come in to see a dentist with a problem. A person with a fracture, swelling, bleeding or pain generally provides a teachable moment (if fear does not immobilize them). Dentists can help clients change destructive behavior more easily when they give feedback that is closer to the traumatic event. A person comes in with a painful abscessed tooth, because they want the dentist to relieve the pain. After their felt need of eliminating the pain is solved, the dentist has an opportunity to give them feedback about what they can do to prevent this problem from occurring in the future. If the dentist waits to talk about how they can prevent a similar problem until the clients next recall appointment, their chance of success diminishes.

2. *It is personal and noncomparative.* Learners need continuous opportunities to have feedback that is personally relevant to their own experiences, to confront new experiences and relate these new experiences to past ones. These opportunities for feedback help them incorporate these experiences into their own lives.

   Comparisons create a hierarchy that places the learner in better than equal to or less than categories. The learner concerns himself more with where he is in relation to others than in learning what is personally relevant for him. People vary widely in their past experiences and the speed with which they learn. People perceive the world differently. Comparisons usually serve as blocks to learning, because apples are usually being compared to oranges.

   In helping clients change destructive behavior, dentists need to find a common ground and set of understandings with clients, and then without comparison, help the clients develop steps to change their behavior.

3. *It is directly related to the task being experienced.* In dental school, I learned anatomy, physiology, bacteriology, biochemistry and histology independent of a relevant task or problem. When I started working with clients, I did not remember what I had been taught in those areas and had to relearn it in relation to the current task. For example, when learning biochemistry, I had no direct experience with a client's problem of converting the foods they ate into energy. There was no immediate patient problem to relate the

knowledge I was learning. If there is an immediate problem, then the learning of knowledge as it relates to this problem is retained better than knowledge learned abstractly.

4. *It points the way to the next steps.* To learn, we need to have a sense of vision or direction. Feedback is of no value if it does not help the learner see what needs to come next. If a dentist says to a client, "you have gums that are red, swollen and bleed easily," without giving them a sense of what they can do to correct the problem, then the dentist is not helping the client solve the problem.

Maslow Hierarchy of Needs

The greatest challenge in helping others learn is when they do not recognize that they have a need to know or learn. An example in dentistry is: when a client comes in with an unrecognized problem such as a missing tooth that is contributing to periodontal disease or is creating a malocclusion. They do not recognize the need to correct the problem with a properly designed bridge. Another example, is presenting the idea of lifestyle change when the client is unaware of how his lifestyle is contributing to periodontal disease.

Abraham Maslow's hierarchy of needs is usually cited as an example of how needs enhance or block learning. Maslow wrote that human needs occurred in the following ordered hierarchy:

+ Physiological needs for air, water and food.
+ Safety needs for security, freedom from fear, and stability.
+ Belongingness and love needs—for affection, a sense of belonging and a sense of being loved.
+ Esteem needs for self respect, self esteem and the esteem of others, competence and achievement.
+ Self actualization needs for self fulfillment and transcendence to actualize potential.

In Maslow's hierarchy, people's basic needs must first be reasonably met before they can give much attention to the higher needs. This hierarchy sheds some light on how people's needs enhance or block their learning. Dentists in the early stages of their relationships with people, primarily help them with physiological needs. Clients have fractured a tooth, have an infection, have facial pain or have a malocclusion. If the dentist attempts to address higher needs, like the concept of wellness or the need for a comprehensive exami-

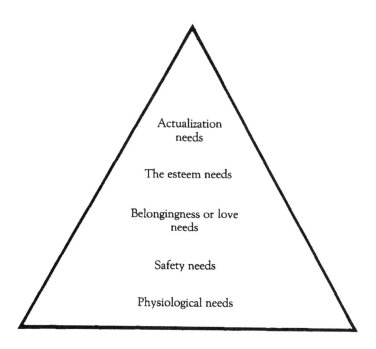

Figure 2. Maslow's Hierarchy of Needs

nation, when the client has physiological pain, the client will not be open to learning about these needs until their pain, disease or illness is resolved. They will be more open to meeting higher needs, such as wellness, after these physiological needs are satisfied.

When a person is in pain, their main concern is relief of the pain, not how much it will cost. If money is an issue in their life, they will be concerned about the cost of treatment when the pain subsides. If money is not an issue, they will be concerned about preventing recurrence, because the pain hindered their feeling of belonging or self worth or self actualization.

In my personal experience, pain and perception of a threat of physical illness can plunge a person from the higher realms to the base of the hierarchy where they are concerned about the satisfaction of their physiological need for health. The client goes from being self-actualized to feeling very vulnerable and frightened. The attitudes of caring, respect, empathy and kindness are particularly valued when a client is in pain or feels threatened by his illness or disease.

When a person has pain, illness or disease, their primary need is to eliminate the pain. After the pain is eliminated, they want to know what they can do to avoid or prevent the pain of the disease from recurring. After this need is met, they will be more open to satisfying the level of need they were at before the event that precipitated the pain, illness or disease. When I first became interested in holistic health and wellness, I had a born again fervor and introduced these ideas to people no matter what was going on in their lives. I failed miserably in helping them to move to an understanding of and commitment to wellness by inappropriately introducing these ideas at the wrong time. I was not relating to them at their level of need.

The following example may help in clarifying the process of learning for a client. Most people make the mistake of assuming that the conveying of knowledge will lead immediately to a change of behavior in a person.

Often a client will enter your practice without any knowledge of a problem. He is not aware of the need to change destructive behavior. An examination makes him aware that he has a problem—for example, periodontal disease. You provide him with information about how the presence of certain bacteria produces toxins that cause the breakdown of his periodontium. You do this sensitively, as you are observant for cues of the clients' feelings, emotions and values. Are they responding with a need to know? With apathy? With indifference? Do they seem threatened, or do they seem to want to know more about what can be done to control the disease?

People Learn Best When They Have a Need to Know

People learn best when they have a need to know and when the event has personal meaning for them. This awareness begins the client's process of learning. He has a need to know how his disease occurred. Information is of little value until the client perceives its relevance to satisfying his personal need of eliminating the pain or disease. Information is valued by the client when he is aware of how it affects his self interest.

The client compares the information against his own experience. "Does what you are recommending make sense to me? If I have a scaling and planing and watch my diet will my gums stop bleeding?" If the information checks out, then the client self-discovers that what you are saying will work for him. This self discovery leads to his making a commitment to learning the self care techniques to control his periodontal disease and to the treatment you recommend.

It is at this point that the client takes action and begins to change his behavior. He begins the self care procedures to change his lifestyle and schedules the appointment for periodontal treatment.

To do the periodontal treatment the dentist has collaborated with the client as a facilitator of learning. He has been sensitive to the client's feelings, concerns, beliefs and values. He has used his knowledge of how people learn to help his clients make informed choices about his dental treatment. The dentist has used the common threads of learning: respect, caring, prizing, understanding, his belief in the client's ability to learn and grow, to help the client make informed choices that will help him change destructive lifestyle habits and to control or eliminate the disease. Often the client's feelings of self worth, self respect, wellness and caring for himself will be enhanced because of his relationship with you and your dental team. Significant learning, growth, healing and change occur because of the presence of the dentist's facilitative beliefs and his facilitative relationship with his client.

Beyond doing dental treatment, dentists need to function as teachers and counselors to enable their clients to learn about and cope with the myriad factors that contribute to dental disease. They are in the behavior and lifestyle business. An understanding of the role that learning and education play in people's lives is integral to the dentist's effectiveness.

Education is a powerful influence on a person's life. It can help or hinder a person's learning, healing, growth and change. An understanding of the influence of the professional education of dentists will help dentists to learn more about learning.

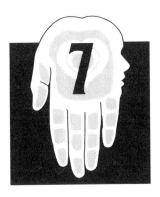

Education

There are two major influences on a person in the first half of life. One is the family environment and the other is his schooling. The educational process is a powerful influence in a dentist's life. This process can help or hinder the dentist's facilitating learning, growth and change in clients. The process by which dentists are educated is a key determinant in their effectiveness in teaching clients to change destructive lifestyle habits.

How dentists have been educated strongly influences the doctor's values and beliefs about people and how they learn. An understanding of the dental school learning environment helps clarify why dentists struggle with the creation of caring doctor-patient relationships.

Much has been written over the years on the educational process and the need for change. It seems that one central function of education should be to help people change and grow. Yet education has been surprisingly resistant to the recognition of this function.

Buckminster Fuller said that there is a 35 year lag time in education between the conception and the application of an idea.

Educational Time Lag

Buckminster Fuller's recognition of a thirty five year lag time is distressingly accurate. It has been approximately that period between humanistic psychology's work on what is an effective learning environment and the adoption of these ideas in professional education.

I have wondered why my feelings about my formal education worsened the longer I was in school. As my education progressed, I felt more manipulated, more coerced, more judged, less understood, less cared for, less respected and less trusted. The low point of my formal education was dental school. It was the most dehumanizing experience of my life.

I remember marveling, "Here I am, a graduate student, soon to become a doctor and I am being treated as less than human. My instructors do not seem to have any experience on how to teach, much less on how people learn. Their only qualification seems to be that they have graduated from dental school or another graduate program. They are repeating the sins of their instructors, who also had no experience or training in how people learn." I was bitterly disappointed that an experience that I had looked forward to, that I had spent countless hours studying to achieve, that my family and I had worked to produce the money to pay for, was the opposite of what I had expected. There was high stress, no trust and no joy, in my dental school experience.

At the time, I thought these feelings were unique to me. They were not. Almost unanimously, dentists relate similar experiences. In an ongoing study, The Group at Cox interviewed 305 dentists and found that in 302 cases, dental school was an unpleasant, demeaning experience for the dentist. Several studies found that from the first year to the senior year there was a decline in the student's self esteem, who became more depressed, more cynical and more distant (Whittemore, 1984, Eron, 1955, Wolf, 1984).

Education as a Process

If education is a process of learning, growth and change, what guidelines are there to support this view? Earl Kelley and Marie Rasey wrote in their book *Education and the Nature of Man* in 1952:

> "At the heart of the business of education is the phenomenon of growth. — If teachers held the concept of growth as the classroom dynamic, it would modify many of their procedures. It might change the teacher himself in regard to his own growth. He would then abandon the idea that children are receptacles, waiting to receive something which he has and they have not. He would see learning as process, and would feel himself to be in the middle of movement, with himself as primary facilitator. He would see that, if the child is to grow, he will have to start where he is, not where the teacher wants him to be, and that the child's progress will have to be measured from that point, rather than from some teacher-measured point."

Dysfunctional Educational Systems

Dental schools are social systems made up of people who interact with each other in much the same way other social groups—families, work groups, church groups and volunteer groups interact. As in these other systems, dental schools can be either healthy or unhealthy systems for the faculty and students that exist within them. I believe most dentists were educated in unhealthy, dysfunctional systems, especially when compared to the environment Kelley and Rasey wrote about in 1952. This dysfunction is passed on through the interactions of dentists with their clients and team members.

Miller's Poisonous Pedagogy

Dental schools have unwritten and unspoken rules and mores of conduct that contribute to this dysfunction just as other social systems do. Alice Miller in *For Your Own Good* has written about the "poisonous pedagogy" of dysfunctional families parenting rules. Miller argues that the poisonous pedagogy is a form of violence that violates the rights of children. This violation repeats when these children become parents. In Miller's "poisonous pedagogy" obedience is valued highest. Obedience is followed by orderliness, cleanliness and the control of emotions and desires. Children are considered "good" when they think and behave the way they are taught to think and behave. Millers' work helps to highlight the poisonous pedagogy that exists in dental schools.

Miller gave the following as examples of such beliefs:

+ Parents deserve respect simply because they are parents.
+ Children are undeserving of respect simply because they are children.
+ A high degree of self-esteem is harmful.
+ Responding to a child's need is wrong.
+ Strong feelings are harmful.
+ Parents are always right.

I am struck by the common beliefs and methods that professional education shares with Miller's examples. Some of these beliefs are:

+ Competition brings out the best in people
+ Students can't be trusted.

+ If it's hard, it's good for you.
+ The punishment of failure helps the person grow.
+ The instructor is always right and shouldn't be questioned.
+ Feelings have no place in education.
+ Students learn at the same rate.
+ Methods are more important than beliefs.
+ Students are not deserving of respect because they are students.
+ All problems can be solved by logic.
+ Students should not make mistakes, and if they do, they should be judged and punished.
+ Perfection is the goal of education.

Student Abuse in Professional Schools

These methods and beliefs are as poisonous to professional students as they are to children. These methods and beliefs result in the doctors assimilating attitudes and beliefs that result in the public's perception of doctors as cold, uncaring, arrogant and autocratic. The sins of the fathers (teachers) pass to the child (student). Going to professional school for the vast majority of dental, medical, naturopathic, chiropractic, podiatry and optometric students is like being raised in a dysfunctional family.

The summary of an article on the incidence, severity and significance of medical student abuse illustrates the problem. "In a survey of the incidence, severity and significance of medical student abuse as perceived by the student population of one major medical school, 46.4% of all respondents said that they had been abused at some time while enrolled in medical school, with 80.6% of seniors reporting being abused by the senior year. More than two-thirds (69.1%) of those abused reported that at least one episode they experienced was of 'major importance and very upsetting.' — We conclude that medical student abuse was perceived by these students to be a significant cause of stress and should be a major concern of those involved with medical student education." (Silver, Henry K. and Anita Dah Glisten. "Medical Student Abuse" *Journal of the American Medical Association* 263 (1990): 527–532).

Why?

How has this dysfunctional system occurred? Why has one of the most important functions of our educational system (the education of health care professionals) become so abusive? One physician called his medical education a scarification process. Why has the work of the pioneers in education (Earl Kelley, Carl Rogers, Arthur Combs) over the last thirty to forty years been ignored? Why does this poisonous pedagogy of the education of doctors perpetuate itself? I do not have the answer to these questions. The answers are involved and complex. Possibly one cause of this abuse comes from the paternalistic, authoritarian and militaristic way that professional school teachers were taught in their schooling. This way of teaching reinforces the poisonous pedagogy that Alice Miller described above.

Learning as an Exciting Experience

I do have a deep belief in the ability of the educators that are in this dysfunctional system to make the changes that are necessary to create an environment in which learning how to care for people is a rewarding, exciting, healthy experience for the educator and the student. I have this deep belief because I feel that learning is inherently joyful, that people desire-even love to learn, change and grow.

A quotation of Alfred North Whitehead was used to introduce another article on medical student abuse in the same January 26, 1990 issue of JAMA quoted above. Whitehead said, "The primary reason for . . . the existence of universities . . . is not to be found either in the mere knowledge conveyed to the students or in the mere opportunities for research afforded to the members of the faculty. Both these functions could be performed at a cheaper rate, apart from these very expensive institutions. Books are cheap and the system of apprenticeship is well understood . . . The justification for a university is that it preserves the connection between knowledge and the zest for life . . . This atmosphere of excitement . . . transforms knowledge. Work . . . is transformed with intellectual and moral vision and thereby turned into a joy, triumphing over its weariness and pain." (Whitehead, Alfred North. *The Aims of Education* London, England: Ernest Benn Ltd: 1932 138–139).

Furthermore, I have this deep belief in the ability of educators to make changes, because I have talked to educators that are trying to change the system, to humanize it from within. I have this deep belief, because the research has been done to show that there is a better way to teach, to facilitate learning. I have this deep belief because there are professional schools who have changed their system and are using the effective principles of learning that I discussed in an earlier chapter in their schools. I have this deep belief because governing bodies like the American Association of Medical Colleges recognizes the need to change.

The student's desire to learn is what has saved the educational system and has kept students from revolting against the tyranny of the educational system in much the way that the American patriots revolted against the tyranny of King George.

If dental education has been a dysfunctional system, what is an effective learning system?

What Is an Effective Learning Program?

Combs' research found that effective learning programs share the following characteristics.

✦ They are tailored to the student's needs, hopes and aspirations. Traditional education, primarily through the lecture process, teaches subjects in an abstract way. The students are not involved in active problem solving. They accumulate information and facts primarily to pass tests. The importance of experiential learning in real life learning situations is critically important. Bob Barkley, D.D.S. said that dentists give clients solutions to problems they did not know they had. Education uses the same approach, by requiring students to accumulate knowledge for problems of which they have no awareness.

✦ They fit the student's experience, values and philosophy.

Effective learning programs provide experiences that are congruent with the student's own life. If the programs conflict with the student's experience, values and philosophy, blocks arise in the student that limit his learning.

✦ They concentrate on the student's belief system, on how he sees the world, and they use the student's perceptions to help him learn new behaviors.

The teacher uses empathy to understand the student's world. This helps the student use his own experience to help him learn new ways of seeing the world or new behavior to learn.

✦ The beliefs of the educator are critical in determining the educator's effectiveness. In the chapter on relationships, I discussed the importance of beliefs (empathy, people as able, self as enough, etc.) in helpers in determining their effectiveness with clients. The same beliefs apply to effective teachers. These beliefs to be effective must be:

1. *Comprehensive.* The broader, congruent and richer the teacher's beliefs are, the more he can help others develop their personal belief systems.
2. *Accurate.* A teacher's beliefs must be as accurate and consistent with reality as possible. This takes us into the area of philosophy and on the tenuous question of what is reality. Yet, healthy people are aware when a person's beliefs are in line with reality.
3. *Internally Consistent.* Since people behave in terms of their beliefs, the presence of internally consistent beliefs gives the teacher a personal security in knowing that his behavior is predictable and congruent with his beliefs.
4. *Personally Relevant.* Abstract beliefs that have no relationship to the teachers own experiences are of no use. If they are not personally meaningful they are not useful.
5. *Appropriate to Problems Encountered.* Sometimes a belief tightly held and narrowly applied keeps a teacher from helping students solve problems. The teacher fails "to see the forest for the trees."
6. *Open to Change.* "There is nothing constant except change." Our life experience gives us feedback to help in reevaluating our belief systems. As we gain experience, we learn more and a result of this learning is more knowledge that may render some beliefs inappropriate.

✦ The educator concentrates on student becoming, rather than "how to." The students are continually involved in personal exploration, the discovery of meaning and the continuous refinement of their personal belief systems. A focus on "how to" contributes to students thinking of their clients dispassionately. Students do not look at the whole of the client's experience, their feelings, personal history and environment. When students learn through personal exploration and the resultant discovery of personal meaning, they learn to help their clients in a similar way.

✦ The educator concentrates on the dynamics that produce behavior rather that the behavior itself. A student may seem
angry, aloof, lethargic. He may not be keeping up. Instead of
criticizing the behavior, the teacher inquires empathically
about what is going on in the student's life. What are the
dynamics leading to the behavior?

✦ The students are expected to take major responsibility for
their own learning.

Traditional education fails miserably in this area. If a student
is going to be helping people become healthier as a doctor,
why not help him become a self directed learner? Upon gradu-
ation, he will be responsible for maintaining his knowledge
of new discoveries. Effective educators help students learn
personal responsibility.

✦ The educator is responsive to students' needs. Students are
not clones. They have different cultural, societal, educational,
familial and intellectual backgrounds. Effective educators are
adept at responding to these differing needs and using them
to help students learn.

✦ The educator is deeply sensitive to students and actively seeks
relationships based on mutual respect and democratic values.
If students are to treat their clients with compassion and
respect, they need to have the personal experience of being
treated with respect by their teachers. Students treat others in
the way they are treated.

✦ The educator facilitates the student's commitment to learning
by exposing them to events and processes designed to create
new needs and to uncover needs they did not know they had.
People learn best when they have a need to know. Creating
needs in students is the greatest challenge to the art of being
a teacher. Seeing the light go on in student's eyes and seeing
them learn in response to your help, is the ultimate reward of
teaching.

✦ Facilities, information and the educator are continually available to the student as the discovery of needs occurs.

The need to know does not occur at pre-ordained times, i.e.,
in the physiology lecture at 10:30 a.m. Monday morning. The
systems of the teaching institutions should be directed toward
what fits, what is good, useful and appropriate for the students
and be flexible in meeting their needs. Traditional education

designs systems for the benefit of the institution and not the student's benefit.

✦ Students explore and discover their own best ways of learning. Research has shown that people learn in different ways. Effective programs recognize these different ways of learning and help students utilize their personal strengths in maximizing their learning.

The "GPEP" Report

Medicine has been the lightening rod for the complaints and criticisms of the shortcomings of health care providers. To its credit, medicine has also pioneered a different healthier approach in the education of its students that meets Combs' characteristics of effective learning programs. In 1984, the Association of American Medical Colleges published a landmark report entitled "Physicians for the twenty first century, the GPEP report." (GPEP is an acronym for General Professional Education of the Physician and College Preparation for Medicine) The report came to five conclusions.

1. The first conclusion "calls for a shift in emphasis among the skills, values, and attitudes taught in medical school: limitations in the volume of information medical students are expected to commit to memory; a better enunciation of the levels of knowledge and skills required at each step in medical education; changes in educational settings; and an emphasis on the responsibility of physicians to patients and communities."

2. The second conclusion recommended that a broad range of activity in the undergraduate education of medical students is recommended to improve writing and communication skills and that these methods be developed to assess analytical skills and capabilities for independent learning, for students applying to medical school.

3. The third conclusion concerned encouraging independent learning by revising the methods of teaching, particularly during the basic science years, by having more unscheduled time in the curriculum, reducing dependency on lectures as the principal method of teaching and providing students with more opportunities for independent learning and problem solving.

4. The fourth conclusion felt that the four years of medical school should be dedicated primarily to the broad and thorough general

preparation of medical students with a more accurate specification of the clinical knowledge and values that are required.

5. The fifth conclusion said that the faculty should be more actively involved in the educational activities of the school. There should be less highly specialized teaching roles, and a high degree of recognition and reward for effective teaching.

The report concluded that medical education should prepare students "to learn throughout their professional lives rather than simply to master current information and techniques—to be active, independent learners and problem solvers rather than passive recipients of information." The report also discussed the importance of selecting students with the "right values and attitudes for medicine and for establishing mentor relationships between faculty and student that model the role of a caring and compassionate physician." This is radical stuff for the governing board of American medical schools to recommend and hopefully will have the same impact on medical education that the Flexner report did in the early 1900's, and surprisingly the "GPEP report" may redress the impact of the scientification of medicine that was a result of the Flexner report.

The McMaster Approach

McMaster University Medical School in Hamilton, Ontario has been the innovator in changing medical education. The school of medicine at McMaster was inaugurated in 1965. The McMaster catalog describes the objectives and intent of the McMaster programme, "The overriding objective to be achieved is the demonstrated ability to identify, analyze and manage clinical problems in order to provide effective, efficient and humane patient care. Enabling objectives consisting of knowledge, skills, and personal qualities to be achieved are the following:"

> *"**Knowledge**. To acquire and put into practice concepts and information required to understand and manage health care problems."*

> *"**Skills**. To acquire and use the following skills."*

> *"**Critical Appraisal Skills**. The application of certain rules of evidence to clinical, investigational and published data, in order to determine their validity and applicability."*

"Clinical Skills. The abilities to acquire, interpret, synthesize and record clinical information in managing the health problems of patients, considering their physical, social and emotional function. Included is the use of the clinical reasoning process."

"Self-Directed Learning Skills. The abilities to identify areas of deficiency in one's own performance, find appropriate educational resources, evaluate personal learning progress, and use new knowledge and skills in the care of patients."

"Personal Qualities. To recognize, develop and maintain the personal qualities required for a career as a health care professional. Acquiring the authority to intervene in the lives of patients carries with it the obligation to act responsibly."

1. *"Toward Oneself.* To recognize and acknowledge personal assets, emotional reactions, and limitations in ones's own knowledge, skills and attitudes, and to build on one's assets and to overcome areas of limitation."
2. *"Toward Patients and Their Families.* To be able, under appropriate supervision, to take responsibility for the assessment and care of patients and their families."
3. *"Toward Colleagues.* To contribute to productive communication and co-operation among colleagues engaged in learning, research, or health care."
4. *"Toward the Community.* To contribute to the maintenance and improvement of the health of the general population."

These are radical innovations in medical education. The way these objectives are carried out are even more radical. I believe you will see the principles of learning advocated by Kelley, Combs, and Rogers carried out throughout the program. The founders identified how they would like to teach and created a program to fit those characteristics. If I were to design a program for dental schools, I would be hard pressed to improve on the McMaster program.

Several other medical schools are implementing the student-centered, problem based, learning approach. Southern Illinois, University of New Mexico, Tufts and Harvard University are schools in the U.S. that are in various stages of carrying out this approach. Schools in Egypt and Holland are beginning programs.

Another innovative program in medical education is the Human Dimensions in Medical Education (HDME) that was founded in

1972 by Orienne Strode. Strode states, "HDME was founded on the premise that in recent years medical science and technology have grown at a faster rate than have the human relations skills of the people who make use of them. Physicians and other health professionals are often seen by their patients as lacking in empathy, counseling and basic human understanding: skills that heretofore formed little part of the teaching in medical education. HDME is a national non-profit education center that is devoted to the improvement of relationships between faculty members and students. Its programs have served several thousand medical school faculty, medical students, and physicians in private practice, often along with their husbands or wives."

This program helped to plant the seeds that has led to the dramatic changes in the thinking of medical educators. HDME is a part of the Center of the Studies of the Person and has been influenced by the work of Carl Rogers and the other members of the Center.

Innovations in Dental Education

In dental education, the University of Missouri at Kansas City, the University of Minnesota, the University of Connecticut, the University of Washington, and the University of the Pacific are making changes in humanizing dental education. In post graduate dental education, The L.D. Pankey Institute for Advanced Dental Education has implemented many innovative approaches to learning.

In dentistry, The Bob Barkley Foundation was established in 1982 to perpetuate the mission Bob Barkely began in the transformation of dental education through humanizing dental education. The Bob Barkley Foundation has worked with dental educators to help them develop more student and client sensitive approaches and to help the students and faculty to become more interpersonally sensitive. This has been done through financial grants to dental educators and experiential workshops in interpersonal relations for dental educators, team members and practicing dentists.

Paulo Freire, a Brazilian educator, said, "changing education is like trying to move a cemetery." I have been impressed with the dedication and sincerity of the dental educators I have worked with through the Bob Barkley Foundation. In the face of some faculty member's resistance to any change, they are committed to making the necessary changes in dental education to create a more humane, effective and responsive environment for dental students and faculty.

It is my hope that the problem based, student-centered approach will continue to expand and the autocratic, teacher-centered approach will become extinct. It is an exciting start.

These programs will help end the abuse of students and enable the students that graduate to create caring doctor-patient relationships and to create humane learning environments for their clients. They will also be well prepared to meet the needs and demands that the twenty first century will bring.

As Kelley and Rasey stated, "the heart of education is the phenomenon of growth" and "the business of teaching is communication." The heart of communication is the ability to listen with real understanding to what the person is trying to communicate.

Author's Note: I realize I have used strong language in this chapter about dental education. I have struggled with whether to include this chapter in this book. I am highly critical of the traditional ways dental students have been taught. Also, I was concerned that this chapter was not about the doctor-patient relationship, because it focuses on the education of the doctor. But, how a doctor is educated is a powerful determinate in how he relates to his clients and patients and how he helps or hinders their learning. I have included this chapter because I feel it is vital that the doctor understand the legacy of his dental education. This is a key to helping him help his clients (and himself) learn, grow, heal and change. I also want to acknowledge that changes toward a more humanistic environment are being made by many individuals and schools in dental education.

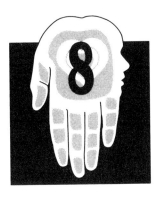

Listening

Learning, growth, healing and change most often occur in clients when I can listen with real understanding and catch the deeper meaning of what the client is attempting to convey. Occasionally, I can help the client recognize what has been unconscious. I feel a great sense of accomplishment when I can catch empathically the deeper meaning of what the client is trying to convey. When I understand their deeper meaning, something happens within the client. It can be as simple as a nod of their head that you caught what they were trying to say, or it can be a welling of tears of gratitude for your understanding of them in a way that few people have.

There is a bias in the traditional doctor-patient relationship against this type of listening or relationship with patients. There is a recognition that communication is important in dealing with patients, but this communication is usually communication to patients not with patients. Webster's Dictionary supports this view. It defines communication as the act of transmitting information. This definition does not catch the flavor of what I want to convey. What I want to convey is more than transmitting information, speaking to a person, trying to persuade, inform, convince or talk to another person. It has more to do with the root meaning of communication—to commune, to make common, to share. Ah, that is it, the key to a caring doctor-patient relationship is communion; an act of sharing, or possession in common; participating—an intimate relationship with a deep understanding of the client.

Dentistry Involves Intimacy

Does the word intimate disturb you? We were taught or more likely it was modeled by dental school instructors that dentists should not get close to their patients. It was not a professional thing to do, patients would not respect us. They would take advantage of us. Now I am suggesting that a key element in communication be to commune with clients—to create an intimate relationship of deep understanding.

Dentists are intimate with their clients. In treating the mouth, dentists are working in a very intimate area of the body. Dentists poke, probe, spray, drill, extract, reduce, cut and curette in this sensitive area that is the clients' primary means of expression and nourishment. Through the mouth, the client expresses joy, sadness, and anger; he speaks, sucks, smiles, curses, laughs, kisses, licks, tastes, eats, spits and drinks. By working in this area, the dentist is automatically intimate with his clients. Denial of the presence of this intimacy and the therapeutic distancing by the dentist from the patient or client is a major contributor to the uneasiness that dentists and clients feel in the dental encounter. The denial of this intimacy results in the crude dental jokes and cartoons that dentists are the butts of; it results in the "I hate dentists" comments and contributes to the dentist's stress and burn out in their profession.

The denial of this intimacy by doctor and patient may result in the overt and covert hostility toward the dentist that was referred to in Chapter 4. These encounters with overt or covert patient hostility can leave the dentist feeling wounded. Often the dentist does not connect the feelings of being wounded—stress, depression, anger, hostility toward patients, team members, himself or family members- with his treatment of patients.

Because of the intimate nature of dentists' relationship with clients and the potential for psychological harm to the patient and dentist, listening with deep understanding is foundational to a caring doctor-patient relationship. This type of listening and interaction between doctor and patient helps to establish trust in the doctor/patient encounters and helps to defuse or alleviate the drama and destruction that overt or covert patient hostility creates for the doctor and patient. Listening with deep understanding helps both the patient and doctor move from constantly coping and reacting to the stressful dynamics that a doctor-patient relationship can create to a more satisfying relationship for both the doctor and patient in which they can create an environment that facilitates healing.

Empathy—What It Is, What It Is Not

This way of listening with deep understanding, of being with another person, is empathy. What does this word mean to me? It means that I can enter the world of my client and move around in an attempt to see how the world seems to him. I lay aside my judgements and my perceptions as I attempt to gently and delicately catch his meaning. It includes giving feedback to my client on my sensings of his meaning, to see if this sense is correct. I respect his separateness. I am a companion on his journey while we are together. I attempt to understand his feelings and problems. I am not able to be empathic to the same degree with everyone. There are days and clients with whom I am more effective, more empathic.

Empathy is not taking the client's problems and feelings into one's own being. It is not to be confused with sympathy. When a helper takes some client's problems and feelings as his problem, this is unhealthy for both the helper and the client.

Active Listening

On a practical level, the ability to listen deeply, which has been called active listening or intentional listening, helps to discover information the client normally would not share with me, but which may have a significant bearing on my treatment recommendations. A client was referred to me with severe headaches for a TMJ evaluation. An examination showed significant wear on the anterior teeth, the presence of an anterior slide and that the medial pterygoid muscle was tender to palpation. Obviously, the client had been clenching and grinding his teeth.

I asked the client if there were any significant stressors in his life. He said "Hell yes, I am going through a divorce." I listened to him as he related how he felt—the fear, anger and hurt he was experiencing. I related to him how I had felt when I went through my divorce. I was empathically with him as he expressed his feelings. I recommended a book and a workshop to him on the process of divorce. The book and workshop had been helpful to me and to several other people.

Besides my normal TMJ evaluation, I had listened to my client and discovered what was going on in his life. Besides the dental treatment for the physical cause of his headaches, I had listened to him with real understanding. This had helped him with the emotional trigger for his headaches. We later heard from the person that referred him, how appreciative he was of how we had listened to and helped him.

This kind of listening can result in the client taking the medication I prescribe, in accepting my treatment recommendations and in following my post treatment instructions. Heszen-Klemens and Lapinska shows that the attempt or orientation toward listening results in an increase in patient compliance and spontaneous health activity.

Empathic listening has a somatic dimension. In the *Language of the Heart*, James J. Lynch's research showed that our "blood pressure is significantly influenced . . . by our capacity to communicate with one another." Lynch worked with his subjects to help them heed what their hearts were telling them by monitoring the rise and fall in their blood pressure. A fall in their blood pressure was associated with speaking less intensely, breathing deeply, attending to others non-defensively and retreating for periods of quiet time. Lynch also said that it was "more important to feel feelings than to control them."

Again, a reductionistic scientific background can make us question the validity and applicability of this way of listening. Philosopher Michael Polanyi had an answer to this problem:

> *"Science is not thus the simon-pure, crystal-clear fount of all reliable knowledge and coherence as it has for so long been presumed to be. Its method is not that of detachment but rather of involvement. . . . in order to understand living things, we must dwell in our subjects of knowledge more deeply—and more deeply yet, as at each step, we seek to know higher animals, until we try to understand the highest animal of all— man. We can succeed here only by a completely reflexive indwelling—a full conviviality with our subject."*

Listening with deep understanding meets Polanyi's description of "completely reflexive indwelling—full conviviality with our subject." It involves active and passive dimensions. Passive listening involves being fully present to the client's meanings, understanding what they mean with their facial and body gestures and expressions, by eye contact, your attentive body posture, nods, Mm's, hums', I see, but it does not include lengthy verbal responses. Active listening includes the behaviors of passive listening and goes beyond these behaviors to provide verbal feedback to your client that "What I hear you saying is _____," "What you feel is _____," "Tell me more about that," are examples of a dentists' intent to catch the meaning behind the clients' word.

Actively Listening

I am concerned about going into the how-to's of active listening. This focus on how to's puts the emphasis on the helper responses and removes the focus from the client. However, I will try to give you a sense of how you can check yourself to see if you are listening with real understanding. David Stindl-Rast, a Benedictine monk, eloquently described the difference between listening with the head and listening with the heart, in his book *A Listening Heart*. "In order to listen with my heart, I must return again to my heart through a process of centering, through taking things to heart. Listening with my heart I will find meaning. For just as the eye perceives light and the ear sound, the heart is the organ for meaning." (1983, 10).

I have found that the most effective way for me to check if I have been listening effectively is to express to my client in my own words what I feel he has been saying. This includes both the verbal content and the feelings that lay just below the surface of his verbal statements. If my client responds with an acknowledgment either verbally or kinesthetically by saying "yes, that is it" or he nods that I have caught his meaning, or he relaxes his body posture, then I have listened effectively. If I receive these validations and the client moves deeper and expands upon what he has said, if he synergistically links seemingly separate thoughts or feelings, if he arrives at a greater understanding or moves deeper; or if my listening evokes a statement or look of gratitude, then listening with real understanding has occurred.

If I have not caught his meaning, he will continue to express what he is trying to convey. He may say "no that's not it, I mean . . ." or he may continue with his description. It has been my experience that when I listen effectively there is a palpable shift in the clients' affect, in his body posture, in his facial expression, in the tone of his voice.

It is common for clients to come to the dentist with feelings of apprehension, anxiety and fear. If we acknowledge these fears with a statement like "It is scary to come to the dentist and have dental work done." The client will respond in whatever way is appropriate for him, and the way is opened to establish a common ground of meanings between the doctor and client. The acknowledgement of their feelings helps them feel more at ease (complete relaxation is usually too much to expect). It helps them when their feelings have been acknowledged and they know the dentist has at least some understanding of what they are experiencing. Alfred Benjamin has described this type of empathic listening as "feeling yourself into, or participating in the inner world of another while remaining yourself . . . to see the world through the (client's) eyes as if the world were his own world." (Benjamin, 1969). The words "as if" are important. If we become enmeshed in the client's world, if we sympathize by feeling an affinity with the person's feelings, we lose our own sense of self by taking into our self the visceral feelings and emotions. We lose our separateness and feel the emotions of loss, fear, anxiety and apprehension of our clients. This is not healthy for the doctor or the client.

Recording the Interview

Recording the interview, either by audio or video tape, is a very valuable tool. Taping interactions with clients and co-workers is an enlightening experience. When I first taped my conversations with my clients, I was appalled at how I sounded (like a hick with a monotone), what I said and how I said it. I was amazed at how much I talked, how much I interrupted, how much I explained, how I jumped in too soon, at what I said or the client said that I forgot and what I missed. Once I worked through the shock, I could listen to how the client was responding to my attempts at communicating. I periodically tape my initial interviews with my clients. I also tape my interactions with clients as I do dental treatment. Taping the general background of the dental office is also enlightening.

I ask my team members to tape their conversations with our clients. There is an initial resistance to or fear of listening to how they sound on an audio tape or look on video tape. If they can go beyond this fear, there is a wonderful opportunity to learn from taped conversations with clients.

It is important to focus on how the client responds to active listening. How do they respond to feedback, questions? Do they accept the feedback as capturing the meaning they are conveying? Do they move and expand because of your feedback? It is natural to focus on how you look and sound on tape. If you only listen to yourself, you will lose the opportunity to learn from the client's perspective how effectively you are listening. Place yourself in the client's shoes. How does it look from his perspective? Allow yourself to make mistakes and do not invalidate yourself by judging. If you feel unsure of where you are or how you are doing, ask a question or questions to establish a reference point of where you are. Omer Reed's classic statement on listening, "Speak to the obvious, ask a question," explains this well. Active listening is a process of arriving at a common meaning. A part of this process is making mistakes in listening until a common, real understanding of the client's world is reached.

I feel it is important to ask the client's permission before recording the interview. I simply ask by saying, "I would like to record our interview. I find that this helps me check on how I am doing. The tapes will be confidential. Is this OK with you?" Once the interview or work begins, both the client and I forget the presence of the tape recorder. Taping is a very valuable way of self-discovering how effective your listening skills are.

Some Other Questions and Comments

Does this kind of listening take longer? It may seem like one more thing wedged into an already full practice. There are times when it can take longer and there are times when it will take less time than you previously spent interacting with your clients. Usually, when a person feels understood, they will not talk as much. The establishment of trust through the process of active listening is a vital ingredient in the doctor-patient relationship.

Recently, a woman was referred to me for several crown preparations by an organization I do volunteer dentistry for. I had not seen her before and she had not been well referred. She had several fractured teeth. Money was not a problem, but we did not have a common ground of meaning. It took a half and hour for us to sort out what needed to be done. We had not built trust into our relationship, and a consequence of this was we had not arrived at a common meaning. In this instance, I elected not to begin the crown preparations until I had done a thorough examination and co-diagnosis, and we had arrived at a common understanding of her need for dental work.

This contrasts with clients with whom I have established a trusting relationship. The dental problem is the same, but the amount of time to achieve a common understanding for the need for crowns takes much less time because trust is established with the client. This way of listening has saved time for me and has immeasurably added to my enjoyment of practicing dentistry.

I can't help everyone that comes to see me. I miss with some people. If a healthy, doctor-patient relationship is not present, the client is usually better off with someone else. In this situation I usually say, "I don't feel good about the relationship we have and feel it would be better for both of us if you found another dentist." Then I stop and listen. The client may agree and we try to establish a good ending to our relationship or they may say, "Oh no, I don't want to leave." If this is the case we try to work out the conflict.

In these instances, it is important that I own my own feelings and use "I" messages. It is vital that I do not project my perceptions onto the client without first checking them out with him. I may say, "I feel like I am not communicating with you or that you don't trust me. I am uncomfortable with this feeling. Are you feeling the same way?" I have found this type of clearing with a client to be very healthy for both of us. As I have become more skilled in listening, fewer of these situations have arisen.

"I just don't feel comfortable in going into depth with this listening stuff, can other people in my office do most of the listening?" My answer is yes, often other members of the team can do the bulk of the helping and listening if there is a common agreement that this is an important part of the team member's job. Team members may be more effective because of the clients' perceptions of the dentist as "the doctor" or the team members may be more skilled at this than the doctor. I had a client tell me that she went to see an OB-GYN because she liked his staff. He was "kind of stiff," but must have been a good physician because of the people that worked for him and the length of time they worked in his office. I feel it is important that the doctor feels that the role of listening is a vital part of helping people. If he or she doesn't, then it will not become an effective part of their practice of dentistry.

Sometimes there is so much going on in the client's life that the dentist is unable to be of help to them physically or emotionally. There is so much static in their life, that they cannot hear what the dentist is saying or respond to his offer of help. They may be going through the breakup of their marriage or a family member may have a serious health problem, and life events influence the clients's perceptions. This can be very frustrating when the dentist sees a dental problem that needs treatment but is unable to help them because of what is going on in their life.

The reverse of this is also true, there may be things in the dentist's life that hinder or prevent his helping his clients. When I went through my divorce, the quality of my relationships, my judgements and my work suffered. I was not as effective in my listening skills or dental treatment.

The congruence of the doctor's actions and words with his feelings and beliefs is essential. Often, the person-centered approach is confused with just being nice to people. It is much more than just being nice, especially if the niceness is a veneer that is unauthentic. There is nothing that turns people off more than phoney niceness or caring. This unauthentic niceness is viewed as highly manipulative. Rogers emphasized the importance of congruence with the helper's actions and words being congruent with his feelings and beliefs. Listening with real understanding is not just being nice to people. It is much more; it includes facilitatively moving people to action, setting goals, challenging and confronting.

Challenging and Confrontation

Making clients aware of needs they did not know they had is one of dentistry's greatest challenges. For example, as a dentist I have many ways of helping people reach an optimum level of dental health in which they will need to have little or no dental work done. To do this, I will need to help my clients become aware of the dental needs they did not know they had. A common example is: a client has been missing a lower first molar for several years. A dental examination reveals that there is Code 2 periodontal disease with a slide from centric relation to centic occlusion and the presence of a working interference on the distal buccal cusp of the second molar in the arch with the missing tooth. There is also crepitis in both Temporomandibular joints.

The dentist sees the need for periodontal treatment, possibly occlusal therapy and a fixed bridge to correct the problems. The client has been unaware of these problems and because he has not had pain, he does not see any need for treatment. "The tooth has been missing for a long time and it doesn't hurt, why should I get it fixed?" The dentist faces a classic dental challenge. How does he make the client aware of needs he does not know he has. How does the dentist challenge and confront the client and help him have the necessary treatment done?

At this point, it is important to distinguish between wants or values based dentistry and needs or disease based dentistry. In an earlier chapter, we discussed Maslow's hierarchy of needs and how the basic needs are gratified before higher needs can be addressed. Threats to the physical self are powerful motivators. The function of swelling, bleeding and pain is to signal to a person that something is out of balance and needs to be corrected. When a client has a painful abscessed tooth his main need and motivation is to relieve the pain. He will cancel all other obligations, trips and appointments to have the pain relieved.

Swelling, bleeding and pain will motivate the client to seek treatment. In needs based treatment, once the problem that caused the swelling, bleeding or pain is solved the patient has no motivation to seek further dental treatment. The motivation to make changes in the lifestyle behaviors that led to the swelling, bleeding or pain disappears with the pain. In needs based treatment the patient is only interested in urgency, crisis care or remedial dentistry that corrects the diseases that led to his swelling, bleeding or pain.

Beyond Crisis Care

In wants or values based dental treatment, the focus is on treating the crisis and doing the remedial care needed to satisfy these lower needs. In addition, values based dentistry helps the client with their higher needs to help them value the more abstract nature of dental health and wellness. For example; self-esteem and self-actualization, what it feels like to be vigorously and abundantly well. To exercise and manage the stress in their life. To have the finest and best dentistry done to help them achieve a lifetime of optimal dental and oral comfort, function, health and esthetics. To eat well so they receive the optimum balance of nutrients to prevent periodontal disease or dental caries.

Dentists have the educated vision and insight to know that unhealthy lifestyle behavior lead to health problems. Most dentists want to do more than provide crisis or needs based treatment. They want to help their patients prevent dental problems by helping them learn how to care for themselves and to live healthy, fulfilling lives.

In the past, dentists have tried to motivate patients to change destructive lifestyle behaviors by preaching, moralizing, threatening, coercing or by being nice and progressively giving in. When this failed, they gave up in frustration on helping their patients change destructive lifestyle behavior. These approaches have not worked well and have led to considerable frustration in the practice of dentistry. In this traditional approach, dentists often feel like nags or adversaries in trying to convince a patient to do something for themselves that the dentist feels is good for them. If people have a basic drive for health, why is it frequently so frustrating to help them become aware of the need for the periodontal treatment, occlusal and restorative treatment mentioned in the example used at the start of the chapter?

Surprisingly, in situations where clients do not place a priority on their dental health, dentists need to negotiate for the basic drive toward health to emerge in the client. In the previous chapters, I have discussed the principles of establishing caring doctor-patient relationships and how these principles are foundational in helping clients learn, change and grow. There are times when a dentist needs to challenge and confront clients to help them change destructive lifestyle behavior and to have dental work done that will help them experience maximum dental comfort, function, health and esthetics.

Challenge and Threat

Combs believes learning and change have two dimensions. One is the discovery of new information or experience and the second is the discovery of the personal meaning of the information and experience. Dentists do the first dimension—the dispensing of new information—well. It is in the second dimension of the client's discovery of the personal meaning of the information or experience that dentists have not done well.

The dispensing of information produces temporary awareness. In dentistry, this has passed for learning. Unfortunately, the dispensing of information does not produce a change in behavior or the discovery of personal meaning. Combs points out that there is a vast difference between knowing and behaving. He says that knowing comes from acquiring new information. Change in behavior comes from the discovery of personal meaning.

Challenge and threat are in the eye of the beholder. Challenge evokes a response toward learning, growth and change. The perceptions of threat causes a person to withdraw, protect, avoid or ignore the opportunity to learn. When challenging, the perception of threat must first be reduced. A threat can result in the changing of specific behavior. In the previous example of an abscessed tooth, the threat of another abscessed tooth may result in the scheduling of an appointment to be sure that there are not other teeth that will abscess. Behavior change from a threat is highly specific and focuses on avoiding negatives and learning what not to do.

Long term learning, growth and change result from the client feeling challenged by the problem. This feeling of challenge enables the client to draw on their resources as they seek to achieve the higher needs of health and well being. Challenge results in more global change and personal affirmation and self-respect. The transformation of a threat into challenge occurs in the safe and freeing atmosphere of a caring doctor-patient relationship.

Confrontation

There are times when the client does not see the necessity of changing destructive lifestyle behavior or of having dental work done. The dentist has done all he can to help the client learn, grow and change in a caring doctor-patient relationship. He has tried to transform a threat into challenge. The client still does not want or does not see the need for changing behavior or for having the dental work done.

At this point, the dentist faces the decision of confronting the client to create a wise agreement. Confronting does not mean a showdown in which someone wins and someone loses, as in an old western gunfight. Confronting is not an attack, is not punitive and is not a fight. The goal of confronting is to help the client learn, grow and change without diminishing their self-respect. In this instance, the goal is to create a wise agreement that helps the client change destructive behavior. This confrontation is done by keeping the client's hopes, concerns and values in mind. The change in destructive behavior enables the client to have dental work done that will optimize their dental comfort, function, health and esthetics and to reduce costs long term.

Confrontation is an extension of the helping relationship. At its best it helps the client see the discrepancies between the value he places upon his health and the choices he makes in relation to his health. For example, the client may say that he wants to improve his dental health. A question we ask the new client in our initial interview is: "On a scale of 1–10 with 10 being excellent, where do you rate your dental health now?" Then we ask, "Where do you want to be?" If the client said that his goal is to have excellent dental health and he has declined to have needed dental work done or to change destructive life style behavior, we confront him with the discrepancy between his stated goal of excellent dental health and his decision not to have the dental work done that would help him attain excellent dental health.

A Breakfast Confrontation

The following is an example of confrontation and negotiation with a client who has periodontal disease and has destructive lifestyle habits.

Dentist   Sandy, you have said that you want to control your gum disease and want to prevent future problems? Have you considered the impact that not eating breakfast has on your gum disease?

Client   I don't like breakfast.

Dentist   You aren't a morning person?

Client   All I can do is drink a cup of coffee and eat a donut. I don't like eggs or bacon and I don't like cereal and all that other stuff.

Dentist   So for you, just getting up, dressed and getting to work is a major challenge. The thought of fixing breakfast is just one thing too many in the morning.

Client   No, I get up all right. I just don't like the breakfast foods.

Dentist   Yet you want to control your gum disease and prevent similar problems from happening in the future.

Client   Well . . . yes.

Dentist   Do you know that gum disease and your diet are closely linked?

Client   I think I may have heard of that.

Dentist   Several experts feel that not eating breakfast contributes to gum disease.

Client   Oh, really?

Dentist   Yes — It seems we have a problem, you don't like breakfast; you have gum disease and want to control it and prevent future problems and not eating breakfast contributes to gum disease.

Client   Yea. It's a problem.

At this point, there is a pause with silence as the client and dentist ponder the problem.

Dentist   Would you be interested in hearing what some other people have done with a similar problem?

Client   Well . . . yes.

Dentist   Some people have made a nutritious shake the night before, so all they have to do is open the refrigerator door and pour the shake in the morning. Others don't like the traditional breakfast so they eat what they would have for lunch or dinner.

Client   I had never thought of that.

Dentist   There is a saying, "You should eat breakfast like a king, lunch like a prince and dinner like a pauper." Maybe you could eat what you have for lunch or dinner at breakfast.

Client   I usually have a taco at lunch. I think that it is good food. It has meat, lettuce, tomato's, cheese and a shell.

Dentist   Maybe you could have that for breakfast.

Client   That seems somewhat strange eating a taco for breakfast.

Dentist   I feel it is important to have breakfast, if you are going to control your gum disease. You probably will not completely control it if you don't eat a nutritious breakfast.

Client   I see what you mean.

Dentist   Would you be willing to try eating a taco or shake in the morning?

Client   I will give it a try.

Effective Feedback

Facilitative feedback is essential in challenging and confronting clients to help them change behavior and have the dental treatments done that the dentist recommends. In the chapter on Learning about Learning, the importance of facilitative feedback was discussed. Combs' work on facilitative feedback was reviewed. Feedback that is maximally useful fulfilled the following characteristics:

+ It is immediate as possible.
+ Is personal and noncomparative.
+ Is directly related to the task being experienced.
+ It points to the next step.

Use Combs' criteria to evaluate the example of a "breakfast confrontation and negotiation."

Motivation and behavior change are challenges to both the dentist and client. There are occasions when the dentist needs to be tough as he challenges and confronts the client. The dentist needs to be tough in the sense that he stays with the client through the difficult process of trusting the client's basic goodness and their basic drive toward health.

This process often includes giving feedback and negotiating with the client to help this drive to actualize.

Roger Fisher and William Ury, in their book *Getting to Yes*, provide some helpful guidelines on negotiating. "Any method of negotiating may be fairly judged by three criteria: It should produce wise agreement if agreement is possible: It should be efficient and it should improve or at least not damage the relationship between the parties." Fisher and Ury define wise agreement as "one which meets the legitimate interests of each side to the extent possible, resolves conflicting interest fairly, is durable and takes community interests into account."

Eight Integral Areas in
Challenging and Confrontation

The following are areas I believe are integral to the process of challenging and confronting.

> Beliefs of the helper
>
> Beliefs of the client
>
> Wants and needs of the helper
>
> Wants and needs of the client
>
> Creating a common ground
>
> Creating wise agreement
>
> Health planning
>
> Action steps

Figure 3.

Beliefs of the Helper

The beliefs the dentist holds create the foundation to his approach to challenging and confronting. A positive view of the client and a belief in his drive toward health is essential. If there is not a belief in the client's drive toward health, the outcome of challenge and confrontation is problematic. A positive view trusts the clients' resources in responding to the challenge of his health problem.

The intent of the dentist in the doctor-patient relationship provides a source from which springs the potential for the client to heal. An intent by the dentist to help the client heal and grow is essential.

Beliefs of the Client

The client's beliefs in himself and in his ability to heal is important. Do they see themselves as trustworthy, as able, as having the resources to heal? What are their beliefs about health care or about the process of healing? Does the dentist understand their beliefs from their perspective? Does he use this understanding to help them make informed choices in their health care decisions?

Wants and Needs of the Dentist

Has the dentist clarified what his values are in relation to his role as a doctor? Does he know how these values create wants and needs in him and in his practice of dentistry? Is he able to communicate these wants and needs to the client in a facilitative way? The dentist wants to help the client become optimally well; To achieve maximum comfort, function, health and esthetics. The dentist values dental health and wellness. These are values that are important to him. These values create certain wants and needs that he seeks to satisfy from his practice of dentistry. When the dentist violates these wants and needs, he does not feel fulfilled in his practice of dentistry.

Wants and Needs of the Client

What are the wants and needs of the client? Does he place a higher priority on other areas of his life than on his dental health? L.D. Pankey felt that 90% of the dental population did not value fine dentistry. Their wants and needs were for a new car, new furniture, vacations, etc. What kind of health care values does the client have? Have they been clarified? Are their actions congruent with their professed values? Can the dentist understand and reflect back to the client his understanding of his wants and needs?

Creating a Common Ground

If there is a discrepancy between the beliefs, values, wants and needs of the dentist and client? Can the dentist create a common ground where both the dentist and client can seek a path in which both of their wants and needs can be met? In a doctor-patient relationship, the interests of the doctor and patient are usually the same—to solve and treat the clients' problems—but often they have different wants, needs and desires.

Creating Wise Agreement

In the dentists case, his interest is in solving the client's health care problem. He has a wider frame of reference and can see the contributing lifestyle behavior that led to the dental problem. The client may feel that the problem can be solved independent of any changes in his lifestyle. A common ground needs to be created in order for the dentist and client to solve the problem in a collaborative way. Fisher and Ury's lovely phrase "Soft on the person, and hard on the problem" describes the importance of recognizing the person, his needs, concerns, fears and anxieties before attempting to solve the problem. The common goal is to help the client become healthier. The confrontation and negotiation process, at its best, is a collaborative one that creates a common ground of wise agreement.

Health Planning and Action Steps

Wise agreement leads to collaborative health planning in which the dentist and client plan a course of action that reflects their beliefs, values, wants and needs. This health plan led to action steps the client has chosen to take. In the breakfast confrontation example, the process was slow until a common ground created wise agreement. When a wise agreement was made, the action steps and health planning proceeded quickly.

Clients' Rights

I feel that the client has a right to make the decisions about their own health. Sometimes, clients make choices that I don't feel are in their best interest. I have helped them define their problem, we have looked at their beliefs, values, wants and needs, but we have not reached a common ground or wise agreement. I have done my best to help the client understand the consequences of his decision not to have the treatment done. He still chooses not to have the treatment done. At this point, I have the choice to decide whether I will continue to work with him and hope he will later change his mind or I will ask him to leave my practice in a way similar to what was described in the previous chapter. I feel frustrated when clients make what I feel is a poor choice. Their decisions trouble me, but they have the right to make those choices.

The following quotation has helped me to resolve this problem. Rolling Thunder, a Native American medicine man had this to say:

> *"We know that everything is the result of something and the cause of something else, and it goes on like a chain. You can't just make the whole chain go away. Sometimes a certain sickness or pain is meant to be because it's the best possible price for something; you make that go away and the price becomes greater. The person may not know that, but his spirit knows it." (Rolling Thunder, p. 123, 1974).*

Challenging and confronting are very satisfying when the client changes destructive lifestyle behavior and chooses to have needed dental work done. However, dentists often shy away from challenging and confronting clients because of the fear of alienating them. When challenging and confronting is done in a facilitative way, they enhance the doctor-patient relationship.

There are also times when the client makes what the dentist feels are poor choices. Our training as perfectionists make it difficult to accept what is perceived as failure on the dentist's or client's part. This comes with the territory of working with people. No one is perfect, and sometimes dentists and clients both make imperfect choices.

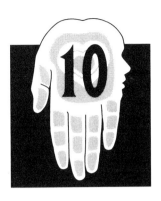

Humanistic Applications in the Private Practice Setting

How is the person-centered approach applied in the private practice setting? In the early to middle sixties, Bob Barkley began developing humanistic approaches to help his clients learn disease control techniques. The process that led to his development of humanistic approaches is an interesting one. Early in his dental career, Barkley discovered that what he had learned in dental school was distressingly incomplete. He initiated a self designed course to correct these deficiencies. He learned from three men, "who made invaluable contributions to my career." From L.D. Pankey, a practicing dentist, he discovered the importance of a philosophy of dental practice and the "Value of fostering a good person-to-person relationship with my patients." From Nathan Kohn, a psychologist, he learned "how to establish such a relationship and then how to educate patients once we had a working relationship." From Sumter Arnim, a research dentist, he learned the importance of controlling dental disease through proper oral disease control measures.

These beginnings led Barkley to discover the importance of a written philosophy of his dental practice, the importance of helping his patients develop a sense of responsibility for their own health, the importance of helping patients develop specific preferred plans for their dental future, the importance of developing a humanistic perspective of management skills, the importance of developing a long term interdependent relationship with his patients, and the importance of helping his patients clarify their health values.

Just before his death in 1977, Barkley wrote in an article titled, "On Becoming a Humanistic Dentist," "I believe that the quality of our upbringing, schooling and religious training have made most of us practicing authoritarians. We must learn to become humanists to the extent of our humanistic potential." He defined humanistic as meaning "A person whose relationship with others is highly inter-dependent, a person whose purpose is to help others to get in touch with their own strengths and develop their own capacities in order to become more effective human beings." He went on to say, "I have only begun. What I have accomplished has drastically changed my self image. If I truly wish to help, I must become more effective in my aid to my colleagues so they can get in touch with their own strengths, values and beliefs. . . . I must try to convince my colleagues to stop frantically searching for answers in the wrong places."

His death at the age of 47 kept Barkley from achieving these goals. I feel Barkley's greatest legacy was in his ability to enable a group of people to catch a vision of a humanistic way of practicing dentistry. He initiated a paradigm shift in dentistry that has been developed and refined over the years into a fully functioning model of a fulfilling and financially rewarding way of practicing dentistry. Barkley's journey of self-discovery led him to the work of human-istic psychologists. His process of learning was like peeling an onion with each layer leading him and the people who followed his teachings deeper.

The person-centered model that has developed includes: human-istic management of a dental practice, a model of self management, team relationships, a participative model of co-diagnosis with the client, whole person approaches, an emerging interest in the spiri-tual dimensions of health care and the concept of a values based practice.

Values Defined

The person-centered approach in dentistry is a values-based process. A definition of a value may be of help. Louis Rath defined a value as something that a person prizes, cherishes and acts upon. When a person values something, he wants more of it—be it love, health, money, nurturing relationships, exercise, good food, under-standing or respect.

Most dentists view their practices from a need driven perspec-tive. Charles Sorenson defines a need as a "feeling you have which you want to be rid of and once rid of do not want again." The old definition of health is the absence of disease. In the traditional medical model, if a patient had a disease they experienced a need to lose it, and once the disease disappeared they did not want it to return.

The person-centered approach includes this dimension and goes beyond to include the values-based aspects of health care. Clients value their health and wellness and want more of it. The clients have personally clarified the value of their health and wellness and seek people—friends and health care professionals—who support them in this quest. The client is interested in curing and preventing disease and in the dimensions of wellness—a group of synergistic approaches that helps a person feel a sense of well being: to feel better physically, emotionally, intellectually and spiritually. Wellness is an ongoing process that emphasizes the generative aspects of a person's life.

Southam's Volitional Practice

Wilson Southam, a dental consultant, futurist, and ergonomic designer, has evolved the concept of a volitional practice to describe a values-based approach to dentistry. With his friend, John Stewart, he has written "A new and powerful model of professional practice is quietly evolving in dentistry. A model which will surely be the pacesetter for all of the health professions over the next decade. Based on a deep respect for the person, this model offers more. More time, more energy, more commitment in support of informed consumer choice. For it has at its heart a commitment to evoking the power of 'volition.' The power in each of us to choose . . . to resolve . . . to will. In the context of health care delivery . . . to choose health . . . to resolve to take care of ourselves . . . to will the requisite new behaviors. Thus, the unstated thesis of volitional practice is: in a health care setting of authentic caring and freedom, most people will choose to strive toward higher levels of self care of their own volition."

Southam and Stewart feel that this values-driven approach provides a more effective level of care to clients, while returning to the dental team a more rewarding and fulfilling way of practicing. The teams who incorporate a volitional approach in their practice have evolved a service model with similar objectives.

Seven Objectives of Volitional Practices

1. To work together as a community of equals whose members are grounded in a shared philosophy and sense of higher purpose.
2. To create a climate of authentic caring and freedom wherein services offered are unadulterated by attempts to control, manipulate or to sell.
3. To take extra time to fully communicate the choices dentistry offers while favoring experiential learning over didactic teaching.
4. To develop the necessary skills of counseling to help clients to create their own health plans.
5. To coordinate the activities of the practice with acute sensitivity to the individual's circumstances, including phasing care to meet the individual's financial and scheduling needs.
6. To offer an excellent cafeteria of self-care supported by hygiene as the foundation of long-term health strategy.
7. To avoid any form of acting, scripting or imitation while striving towards genuine congruence of values and behavior in all walks of life.

The building of a person-centered or volitional practice takes time and is a developmental process. It is a discipline, skill and art that is developed over time. It is not instantly created by imitating others or by quick fixes. Its foundation is a philosophy of care that is based upon personally clarified values that result in excellence of care. This excellence of care is both technical and behavioral. It is challenging to those who choose to implement it as long held beliefs are confronted, clarified and when appropriate changed. For the teams that believe in this way of practicing dentistry, the outcome is a personally and financially rewarding way of caring and helping people.

Perhaps the following letter and article will help describe my journey in integrating the person-centered approach in my life and my dental practice. The first letter is one that I wrote to Avrom and Deborah King and was published in Nexus one year (1977) after the first Dr. Becoming letter was published. The second is an article that was published in Nexus in 1978.

The Second Dr. Becoming Letter

"Remember my participative office? Well, I discovered that it wasn't. When I returned from the Participatory Management Workshop, I really thought and felt that ours was a participatory office. Slowly, I came to realize that I had grossly distorted the facts. (I lied like hell.) I was uneasy in my relationships with my staff, but I didn't realize what was happening until I explained to a friend, a NEXUS subscriber, what I was doing. Here is what I told him: On Monday I was participatory or person-centered. Tuesday I was directive. Wednesday was my day off. Thursday I was authoritarian. And on Friday, I (and everyone in the office) was so confused and frustrated that we couldn't wait for the weekend to start. This obviously produced a lot of stress and anxiety because no one knew who I was going to be. Putting it mildly, I was lacking in genuineness or congruence.

I also came to realize that I had (have?) a strong need to control everything and everyone in "my" office. I literally was Maslow's hammer (ball-peen), and I had pounded many nails. This attitude, and my lack of personal congruence, resulted in two of the three people who attended your workshop quitting. It really hurt me when they quit because I really thought I had a participatory office. Now I think I realize what caused them to quit.

The realizations of how I influence the character and configuration of my practice is both exciting and awesomely scary. The people around me are mirrors and the reflections I see can be disconcerting.

Another insight I have had, is how intensely competitive I am. I was raised in an atmosphere that stressed competition. This competitive attitude was enhanced in dental school (my thing (crown) is better than your thing). I had a need to be perfect, excel. I am a damn good competitor, but competition is only productive when you think you can win. How do you win when you are competing with yourself? I did a lot of comparing with other dentists and people. I drop magic names like Pankey Institute, Reed, NEXUS, etc., etc. I have blah, blah, blah. What a bunch of wind, but I still do it. I hear that so and so did $000,000 last month or year. I did more or less than that. I feel superior or inferior.

The saying "If you see the Buddha on the road, kill him," is becoming very real for me. You know from my other letter that I was searching for the magic solution to everlasting happiness. I found that I was giving my power away by deifying others into super-beings and then depending on them to solve my problems for me. I have killed a lot of Buddhas. But I am the process of learning to trust myself.

Being in touch with my anima-animus (feminine-masculine) has resulted in a freeing of my softer side. My anima helps so much in my people relationships. However, when I am doing the mechanistic aspects of dentistry, I had better be in touch with my animus or I don't finish an equilibration or the bridge won't fit. I frequently have trouble making the instantaneous switch from mechanics to people and then I become frustrated. I have gradually let go of the (hierarchical) doctor-patient relationship, and I am establishing a mutual relationship in which we both can grow. I view myself as a helper and resource person. This has reduced my anxiety more than anything. **The patient is responsible for his health not me!!!** *I very much value the SRI profiling service. I have used it in hiring two people. I now have a receptionist who is a warm, caring, empathic person who hates typing and book work, and an assistant who did not know mesial from distal, but who thoroughly enjoys helping people. But that's all right! We are learning, growing and caring together.*

Well, all this is related to my practice. I want to share with you my personal odyssey and growth. It has been scary, exhilarating, joyous, disconcerting. But it feels great. The journey has been in getting to know, trust and love me—Lynn Carlisle. Truly self-discovered learning. Our friend, Carl Rogers has written: "It is not the special professional knowledge of the therapist, nor his intellectual conception of therapy, nor his techniques, which determine his effectiveness. It is the extent to which he possesses certain personal attitudes in the relationship. They are congruence or genuineness, empathic understanding, and unconditional positive regard." It took a long time for the meaning of those words to sift from my intellect to my gut. I am now, just now, getting a glimmer of what they mean. I was trying to apply empathy, congruence and unconditional positive regard as skill to other people. But it wasn't working. What resulted was apathy, confusion and distrust. **It took me a long time to learn that I had to be empathic, genuine and unconditionally loving with me before I could help others.** *I recognized this long before I felt it. When I experienced this, I started letting go of a lot of perfection crap—trying hard (forcing), controlling, comparing. I became much more accepting of myself, and in accepting* *me; I was able to trust and love myself enough to let the real me show through. Hey! I can be me, genuinely me, and that is much easier.*

I had always avoided confronting (or even getting in touch) with my real feelings. I had expended a vast amount of energy in trying to maintain a facade. I was afraid that a creature from the Black Lagoon was lurking somewhere behind my facade. Through reading, workshops, groups and communities, I discovered that this fear was not valid. Suddenly, previously troublesome things started falling away like ugly scales. People were more accepting of me. The atmosphere in our office became more harmonious. I can let people love and care for me and I can love and care for others, particularly significant others.

I have given myself permission to fail or to do poorly. *Under this condition, miraculously, I don't seem to fail or do poorly as much. I trust the process more and in that trust, good things just seem to happen.*

This was a very inward, self-centered journey in self-discovery. As I tumbled, fought, searched, I forgot about others at times. They felt far away—wife, family, co-workers, friends. At times, it was and still is lonely. I have to have and remember (remind myself) to know and own what I am feeling at the moment, good and bad, so I don't repress it.

My awakening started with the warm, caring nurturing people at a Center for the Studies of the Person "Living Now" workshop. They helped put me in touch with how special people are. (Rereading this tells me that I sometimes lose touch with the value of people. In my last letter, I talked about my discovery of how great people are. I discovered it again. I probably will rediscover it many times.) As you can tell, I still experience stress, doubt, suffering and frustration. But now I view them differently. I think that they can create a positive tension in which growth occurs.

In this workshop, Stanley Keleman diagramed growth this way:

ENDINGS → BEGINNINGS → MIDDLE GROUND → NEW FORMS

He said that before you can have beginnings, you have to have endings. Endings release energy so you can venture forth. This energy sends you into the middle ground which is a place of confusion. Out of this confusion come new forms, new directions. William Blake tells us "That anything capable of being imagined is an image of the truth." It is my perception that is important. When I can focus on an idea, then that idea will become real for me. In moments of confusion, if I can visualize in my mind an idea or goal or hoped-for event, then I can use my creative tension to venture forth. In venturing forth, I feel trepidation, doubt and stress, so I retreat to a safe harbor where all things are known. When the known become uncomfortable and no longer tolerable, then the idea or desire I passionately want seems to happen in a synthesis and wholeness that often transcends the initial goal or idea. It "just happens." Naturally and spontaneously. But everything that had gone before helped create the happening.

The thing I still value the most is relationships. Warm, caring, nurturing, loving relationships. (I'm discovering it again.) This is the harbor, the reward, the renewal-recharger for me. These relationships can just be there, or they can be elusive. So elusive that I wonder if I will find-experience them again. But when I allow this love to flow through me and don't try to grab it or contain it, I become free to start:

> Living beginnings
> Living changes
> Living endings
> Transcending
> And beginning again
> Living Now

> *Gay Leah Swenson*

That helps me to:

> Love, laugh, cry
> Grow
> Feel—snow falls, rain falls, sun glows
> Feel life's rhythms, patterns, transitions
> Hard, fast, easy, slow
> Grow
> Trust and love you
> Trust and love me
> We
> Be. Become all I am meant to be.

> *Lynn Carlisle*

Some Observations on the Dr. Becoming Letters

Carl Rogers has called what I went through (and still am) "a process of becoming." Learning is not a smoothly ascending process. Somehow, we have acquired the ideas that there should not be any setbacks along the path of learning. I remember when I learned how to downhill ski. The first time I went skiing, I knew that skiing was something I loved doing. I went every chance I could. I read books, magazines, brochures, planned trips, looked at equipment, went to ski movies and eventually moved to Colorado so I could ski. I also took terrible falls on easy slopes, hard slopes and everything in between. I broke some skis and became immensely frustrated at my slowness in learning. In rereading my Dr. Becoming letters, I realize that I followed a very similar progression in dentistry. I had an intense interest in helping relationships and the techniques and philosophy that was presented at the L.D. Pankey Institute for Advanced Dental Education. I read voraciously, attended workshops, tried out the approaches presented and made numerous mistakes along the way. Figuratively, I fell down numerous times, made the necessary corrections from my mistakes, and continued on my way to learn more.

In some ways, I am still confronting several of the same issues now and many of the other problems I was dealing with when I wrote the letters, have fallen away. Now, I am much more congruent in my relationships with my team members and clients. I still make mistakes, but they are much less frequent and usually result from my not paying attention to what I am doing. This is also true of where I am technically in dentistry.

The middle 70's were a yeasty time for me as I made major discoveries in my personal and professional life. It was during this time that I progressed through the continuum's at the Pankey Institute, became interested in wellness and holistic health, went to the Center for the Studies of the Person programs, built a new office, and went through a divorce.

I wrote the following article in 1978. It was published in the NEXUS newsletter and describes my interest and experiences in holistic approaches to dentistry.

Cracks/Transformations

At a workshop on facilitation, I recently met a psychotherapist who had been a dentist. He mentioned that he felt part of him would always be a dentist. I asked him why. His reply had a crystallizing effect on me. He said: "An instructor in dental school told me what it would be like to be a dentist. He described it by saying that every time I went by a building, I would always notice the building's cracks and irregularities." That is a heavy statement and it provides a dilemma for the dentists who will become interested in holistic health. It is a direct contradiction for a person who has been trained in the reductionistic, atomistic science of dentistry to practice holistic health. How can a person who has been trained to see cracks (disease) help a person in a holistic way? The answer is simple/complex. It involves the total transformation of your life (not just your dental practice). The transformation is generated by seeing the harmonious whole of a person, with the attendant frailties, strengths, joys and ambivalence, instead of viewing the person as an assemblage of parts, each with its own biological function and physiological dynamic.

A year ago I had what I thought was a revelation. Why not emphasize health, total health . . . instead of disease? With utter naivete, I believed this to be one of the great thoughts of history. Well, it was, but it has been discovered and rediscovered since the dawn of humanity. Its latest rediscovery is going on now. So, holistic health is new/old.

A question I have asked myself is: "Is it (practicing holistic health) worth it?" I believe that for me, it is. But the implementation is difficult, and it indeed is involving the transformation of my life. I have been implementing holistic health in my practice during the past year and would like to share some of my thoughts on dentistry and holistic health.

When I view my function as preventing disease, repairing defects or actively intervening in the disease process, then by this attitude I will probably create or cause more disease or repair than I cure. For example, several recent studies have affirmed that in areas where there are more physicians, there is a corresponding increase in the number of deaths. I think that if lost teeth or edentulous mouths were studied in the same way, dentistry would demonstrate the same phenomenon. I see this becoming more of a problem in the future—as more dentists graduate from dental school. There will be fewer patients per dentist, resulting in practices that are not busy. When a dentist's training emphasizes repair or prevention of disease, he is confronted with a dilemma. How do I earn a living, the good life that I promised myself, if I don't have enough patients in my practice?

This dilemma is exactly the same as the one facing a dental student when he is confronted by the quota system in dental school. "I need 20 units of crown and bridge to graduate. It is April of my senior year, and I only have 15. I will do a crown on a patient who does not need a crown in order to fulfill my needs, not the needs of the patient. Or on a state board, I will look for an incipient lesion that I ordinarily would not restore. I will do a class 2 restoration because of the state board's demand for an ideal preparation, not because it is best for the patient."

When a dentist starts his private practice, the model for ethically dubious behavior has already been established and rewarded. When the rent is due or a loan payment is past due, a conscious or unconscious process tends to favor a procedure which, under different circumstance might not be done. It is the overt, atomistic emphasis by traditional dentistry on repairing and preventing disease that cause this dilemma. I feel the emphasis should be changed from the atomistic procedural focus upon prevention and repair, to a whole person or holistic focus on helping the person become healthier and if the client wishes it, to attain optimum health. When this attitude (holistic) is genuinely believed by the people in dentistry, dentist and staffs, health means more than the absence of disease (which is the current definition of health).

A person can be classified now as normal (or healthy) and that person can still be overweight, smoke, eat junk food, get out of breath after minimal exertion, etc. Is a resting pulse rate in the 70's and 80's healthy? It is now viewed as normal because most people's pulse rates are within that range. Or is a pulse rate in the 40's or 50's healthy? If the emphasis was on health or wellness, perhaps normal would become a pulse rate in the 40's or 50's. I feel that optimum health (or wellness) should be understood and sought by both the client and doctor—if they both value it.

I am not discounting the knowledge and techniques of repair and prevention. The skills of traditional dentistry are, potentially superb. If I were to become injured, have a hereditary problem which needed correction or develop an acute bacterial infection, there is no one I would rather have help me than a person who is competent in treating acute disease or repairing injury. But I would hope that the practitioner's attitude and philosophical orientation is directed toward helping me to return to optimum health—not just resolving the visible manifestation of my problem. I think people in dentistry can do both. But it will require a foundational change in their attitude from the atomistic to the holistic. The omnipresent danger for people who are interested in holistic health is that they will view what is essentially a philosophy, as a series of techniques for making a person whole. The orientation toward techniques is totally incongruent with holistic health, and it will be as deadly to holistic health as it was to the preventive dentistry movement.

I feel that the most we can do is to create a time and place where self-learning can occur. I believe this happens best in a small group in which self-directed learning (or freedom to learn) is encouraged by a facilitator—who may or may not be a dentist. Being a facilitator involves providing resources, a time and place to meet, trusting the process, believing that people have an inherent desire to grow, being empathic, genuine and unconditionally accepting of the people in the group.

I believe the following thoughts are important and that they should be kept in mind when discussing holistic health. I share them with you because they have been helpful to me. I have tried to attribute these thoughts to their authors. But the origin of some of the concepts is obscure:

> *Each person is responsible to self for health. Trust the process.* (Carl Rogers)

> *Health is a question of balance.* (Paul Brenner)

> *Self-acceptance is the beginning of change.* (Carl Rogers)

> *Love is a gift to be cherished and then passed on.* (Lynn Carlisle)

> *Sometimes the magic works and sometimes it doesn't.* (Thomas Berger)

> *Creating a climate of freedom to learn is essential to holistic health. Three key elements of holistic health are faith, exercise and nutrition.* (Lynn Carlisle)

> *It is the integration of the body, mind and spirit that results in a whole that is greater than its parts.* (Unknown)

There is order and meaning to each of our lives. Health and dis-health are in a constant state of flux. Illness is blocked love. (Paul Brenner)

Ya gotta believe. (1969 New York Mets)

Becoming not Being (Carl Rogers)

For a physician to observe chronic illness in a Newtonian cause/effect manner is preposterous. (Paul Brenner)

If you have experienced your wholeness, no explanation is needed. If you have not, no explanation will do. To be a winner, one must be willing to lose. Paradoxes create conditions for learning. (Lynn Carlisle)

Unconditional love is the life force. (Unknown)

Lecture only creates awareness. (Lynn Carlisle)

Life is best understood backwards, but it must be lived forward. (Soren Kierkegaard)

Personally, I'm always ready to learn although I do not always like being taught. (Winston Churchill)

It is important for a man to look to tomorrow and want to carry on, so keep on carrying on. (Jerry Jeff Walker)

People learn when they are ready to learn. (Unknown)

It seems we are exceedingly defensive about our health. I believe this is because the closer something or someone is to a person, the harder it is for that relationship to be open to change—learning and growth. The principle approaches the status of a law of physics: the closer to the center, the harder it is to be free and open. But when a person experiences success in one area of holistic health, there is a natural inclination for growth to begin in other healthful areas. This process is difficult. It involves changing fixed attitudes by growing and stretching. But the rewards of experiencing your own or another person's emerging wholeness is one of life's transcendent experiences."

In Retrospect

I am struck by the themes that I established for the next 15 years of my life during this time. I have spent the time since the 70's learning, refining and expanding on the themes I first explored in the Dr. Becoming letters and the Cracks/Transformations article. The challenge for me has been to integrate these philosophical themes and thoughts into my practice and personal life.

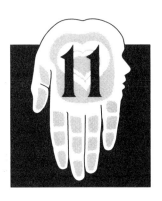

Nitty Gritty Approaches in Private Practice

Recently, a person asked me what was different about the way I practiced dentistry when compared to other dental practices. This question caused me to stop and think about what is different about a person-centered way of practicing. What characteristics would a person see that differentiates a person-centered dental practice from other dental practices? What would a client or a consultant with no experience in a person-centered practice see in a person-centered practice?

After thinking about the question, "What is different?", I replied. "If you came into our practice you would see that we do many things that other dental practices do, but the environment we practice in and our beliefs are different from most practices. You would see that we do many of the same dental procedures. The bulk of what we do is to provide dental care. If a person has swelling, bleeding or pain we take care of that. If a person has gum disease or dental decay we treat that. If a person wants to maximize their dental comfort, function, health and looks we create a plan with the person to do that. If a person wants to prevent dental problems and learn self care techniques we help them learn ways to do this."

What Is Different?

"The things that are different are: our long term commitment to wellness with its emphasis on exercise, nutrition, stress management, and faith: our holistic focus and our belief that a person's beliefs, feelings and spirit influence their physical health, the way we participatively work together as a team, the work we do with chronic disease and chronic pain patients and our relationships with our clients."

Since this question, I have frequently thought about "What is different?" Sometimes, I feel evangelical and even arrogant as I extol the virtues of person-centered approaches. There are significant differences in person-centered approaches. What would the client or consultant see if they went into a person centered practice? Specifically, what systems or nitty-gritty approaches would they see?

They would see:

✦ An emphasis on collaborative team and client relationships.

✦ An emphasis on long term health planning. This long range health planning would occur in a helping relationship to help the client define personal lifestyle objectives.

✦ A focus on wellness instead of just eliminating disease.

✦ A holistic instead of a reductionistic focus.

✦ An emphasis on the creation of a facilitative, learning environment.

✦ A commitment to the personal and professional growth and actualization of the team members.

✦ A focus on the active involvement of the client in their health planning.

✦ A feeling that a caring relationship with the client is as important to the client's well being as the dental treatment.

✦ A focus on participatory practice management.

✦ A commitment to behavioral and technical excellence, to doing one's best instead of perfection.

✦ A belief that pain and disease provide information about conflict and disharmony.

✦ An emphasis on process over achieving end points.

✦ A utilization of alternate health approaches.

✦ A focus on a values based philosophy driven practice.

✦ A focus on service and a belief that out of the service of giving will come personal, spiritual and financial fulfillment.

✦ An openness to change.

✦ A growing recognition and openness to the importance of spirit in their practice.

✦ A belief in the importance of collaborating instead of competing with dental colleagues.

✦ An effort to simplify, to do "more with less" and to go beyond competence to finding meaning and direction from their practice of dentistry.

✦ A recognition of the role of mistakes as part of learning.

Obviously, there is no one practice that exhibits all of the above characteristics. I feel if you went into a practice that was moving toward a person-centered way of practicing you would, over time, see the intent to manifest these characteristics in the personal and professional lives of the dentist and long-term team members.

Integrating the Person-Centered Approach into a Practice

The following are ways that different teams have integrated person-centered approaches into their practices. They fall into the following categories: Philosophy, mission and vision, planning, focus on building a team, communication and marketing, relationships, health therapies and health and wellness counseling.

Philosophy, Mission and Vision

A common theme or characteristic in person-centered practices, is the recognition of the importance of personal and professional clarified values and a development of a philosophy of practice. Without undergoing this process and discipline, dentists are "skilled barbarians" as Steven Muller, president of Johns Hopkins University, said in an interview. His whole quotation is: "The university is rooted in the scientific method, and the scientific method cannot provide a sense of values. As a result, we're turning out skilled barbarians."

A written philosophy statement provides a vision of the highest and best that you strive for and it gives meaning and direction to your practice. The philosophy statement is developed collaboratively by the dental team. A philosophy statement is invaluable as a touchstone to check out the congruence of a dental practice's decisions and systems. It helps the team define the highest and best that are in them, and it helps them to achieve their potential. It is what the team strives for, it is not always attained or actualized, but the intent to achieve it is present in the team.

This is the Carlisle Dental Group's most recent philosophy and mission statement.

Our Vision

Helping People become healthier through our practice of dentistry.

Our Mission

We desire to give the best we have to offer to our clients, while respecting their values, concerns, attitudes and integrity.

Our Group

Our intent is to be responsible to each other and our clients for the ongoing creation of a rewarding, challenging, supportive and enjoyable environment.

Public Service and the World

It is our intent that our services will add value to our community, humanity and our world.

When I first wrote my philosophy statements, they were more a reflection of the most recent presenter I had heard. I wrote them because I was told good dentists did this, and I thought it would help me make more money. Over time, they have evolved into a reflection of my values and philosophy of practice.

Development of a Team

A commitment to a person-centered way of practicing causes many changes in a practice. One of the most challenging is the abandonment of a hierarchical top down style of management, to the development of a collaborative team approach to dentistry. Doug Young describes the hierarchical style of managing employees as the "King/Queen-twit" Model. In this model, the dentist is the King or Queen—the omnipotent authority, an all wise, all knowing leader. The staff members are the "twits." They are the girls, the followers of orders, the paid help that is expected to do exactly as they are told. They are a necessary nuisance to practicing dentistry and are a source of frustration.

Over the years, I realized that the quality of the people I worked with has a profound impact on my own life and those of my clients. The quality of the people and the relationships I have with them directly reflects upon me as a doctor. I discovered that the more I trusted the people I worked with, the more they could be trusted. If I shared the inner workings of my practice—the cash flows, my goals, my hopes, expectations and frustrations—they could be trusted and wanted to help me attain them. I included them in the decisions of the practice: the formulation of the philosophies, mission, purpose and goals of the practice, the hiring of personnel, the making of purchase decisions, the development and refining of practice systems. They became stakeholders, and their participation gave them a sense of ownership in the practice.

Some of the things we have done to implement a team approach in our practice are: we have team meetings for 20–30 minutes before our day begins to discuss the business of the day—who is coming, what we will need, how we are feeling, review our goals, problem solve and plan. We spend one morning a month in a team meeting in which we look at more global issues. For example, workshops to attend, budgeting, equipment purchases, reviewing our philosophy and business plan, planning changes in our office systems, discussing our ways of marketing and sharing our wisdom, caring and frustrations. There are also times of confrontation as individual's actions are challenged if they interfere with the teams and practice's healthy functioning.

Hiring

Another result of the team approach is that we have drastically changed the way we hire people. We have discovered that the person's beliefs and attitudes are more important than past dental experience. If we find someone with values and beliefs that are congruent with the person-centered approach, who has past dental training, we are then obviously getting the best of both worlds. If we need to make a choice, we choose a person who shares common beliefs and values with us, instead of someone who has prior experience. We use a lengthy hiring process that is designed to find a person with beliefs and values that are congruent with ours, who has the aptitude for the job position.

Personal Growth

There is a strong emphasis on the personal growth of the team members and money is budgeted for personal growth classes. Some classes attended are: stress management, therapeutic touch, care for the caregiver, helping relationship classes, assertiveness training, meditation, guided imagery, nutrition, working women's conferences and time management.

Communication and Marketing

We created a newsletter in 1977 to educate the people in our practice about our whole person and wellness approaches. Since then, we have included many topics in the newsletter. These include: dental topics, wedding announcements, copies of wedding ceremonies, reprints of articles, nutrition, exercise, introduction of team members, practice announcements.

The newsletter has become a valuable resource for client information. We have a file of past issues that cover a rainbow of topics. We will mail or give past issues to clients that are appropriate to what is going on in their life. We also maintain a file of reprints from magazine articles that we also send to clients. Similarly, we have a lending library of books, audio and video tapes for our clients. We have developed a series of outreach programs that we present to local business, service, government and church groups.

We have worked with a marketing group to develop service based marketing approaches that are congruent with our philosophy, mission and vision. We have identified what our unique service position is and have developed ways to make the intangibles of the person-centered approach tangible to our existing and our prospective clients.

We do small targeted marketing through groups and publications that we feel are compatible with our philosophical approach to dentistry. We "AFR" (ask for referrals) continually from our clients. Our main source of referrals is from existing clients or other health care professionals (approximately 90%).

Client Advisory Board

We also have created a client advisory board in our practice to give us opinions and direction. It is composed of 12–15 people and meets on an as needed basis. The following criteria are used to make our selections: we like the people, they share common values, they have committed to optimizing their general and dental health, they are a representative cross-section of our practice. The response they have given us includes: the importance of building relationships with them, of being fully present and focused when we do their dental work, the importance of doing technically excellent dentistry, the importance of listening to them and in being gentle and caring. They have also asked how we market, why do we practice dentistry and what business are we in? The client advisory board is one of the most rewarding and valuable things we have done. We are learning of its potential to help us.

Relationships

These activities occur in an environment that emphasizes the importance of caring, helping relationships. This intent permeates all of our activities. Perhaps the best example is how we bring people into our practice.

Bringing a Person into Our Practice

A profound change we have made is how we bring people into our practice in a nonurgency or nonemergency situation. Instead of the traditional examination, diagnosis and case presentation, we use a process developed by Bob Barkley that he called "three phase adult education." This includes the initial interview appointment, the co-diagnosis appointment and the long range health planning appointment. Bob Frazer, Bruce Pettersen, Michael Dick and several other dentists have refined Barkley's work. The following explanation shows the influence of their work.

Initial Interview

The three phase process begins with an initial interview appointment in which we (dentist or team member and client) collaboratively discover the following together. What are the client's needs and expectations about their dental health? For example, we ask, "On a scale of 1–10 with 10 being excellent where would you rate your dental health now?" "Where do you want it to be?"). What are their dental and wellness goals and values? What are their fears and concerns? What is their dental and medical history? During the initial interview, we share briefly with the new person our philosophy of practice and our hopes, needs and expectations of dental practice. We gather the necessary records at this appointment: X-rays, study models, bite registrations, nutritional survey, wellness survey as needed.

Co-Diagnosis

The second appointment is the co-diagnosis appointment. During this appointment, we discover with the client, what is happening with their dental health. (Intra-oral cameras and video imaging technology are valuable tools that help the client participate in the co-diagnosis process.) For example, missing teeth and the problems that occur from the missing teeth, cracked fillings, areas of decay, gum problems, bone loss and malocclusions. We serve as a consultant to the client as we help him think about his present dental condition and what his dental health goals are.

We help the client develop a long range plan for achieving their desired goals and a plan to stay healthy and achieve a state of wellness. The following is an example of how we do this. "Generally people come to see us for one or a combination of the following five reasons (urgent, remedial, complete dentistry, preventive/self care and wellness resourcing). They have an urgent problem; our definition of urgent is if you think it's urgent, it is. They have some remedial problems, some active dental disease like dental decay or gum disease. They want complete dentistry to maximize their dental comfort, function, health and esthetics. They want to learn preventive and self care techniques to prevent future dental problems. They are interested in wellness approaches, especially about exercise, nutrition and stress management.

Health Planning

The client responds to one or more of the five areas and then we do the final phase with him of health planning which involves: selecting the treatment to be done, the period in which it will be done and arrange payments. (Bob Frazer, D.D.S. has an excellent video tape on the three phase examination process. The address is 8118 Shoal Creel Blvd., Austin, Texas 78758. The phone number is 512-454-5743).

The following outline summarizes this process.

Initial Interview

Intent: Initiate long term collaborative relationship and problem clarification and create an environment that helps people feel empowered and safe.

Helper Activities: Listening, warmth, caring, respect, empathy, congruence and genuineness. Discover what the client wants and feels is relevant. Become aware of the needs and values of the client.

Client Activities: Self-exploration, value clarification (health), understanding where the client thinks he is dentally and where he wants to be.

Specifics: Personal history, medical history, dental history, necessary X-Rays, study models and take care of any urgencies.

Co-Diagnosis

Intent: Continue to establish long term doctor/patient/client relationship. Help the client explore, examine and set goals based upon the client's dynamic understanding of the co-diagnosis process. Help the client identify where he wants to be using the long range health planning concept. Also, to help the client understand what will likely happen if they choose to do nothing.

Helper Activities: Discover where the client is and why he is the way he is. (Clinical examination) What is needed to achieve where the client wants to be in the future. (Health Planning) Help client become aware of needs and wants he did not know he had. (Promoting new health and dental perspectives) Give feedback to client on his choices, and help him set his dental health and wellness goals.

Client Activities: Develop new health perspectives. Set health, wellness and dental goals based upon a dynamic understanding of his dental health. Understand the need for acting on the goals that have been set.

Specifics: X-Rays, study models, information from initial interview appointment, mirror, explorer, periodontal probe, intra-oral camera for oral/dental examination. We also palpate the muscles, TM Joint and the teeth.

Long Range Planning and Consultation Appointment

Intent: How to become and remain healthy. Creating action steps (Treatment plan)

Helper Activities: Want to do dentistry under the best of conditions instead of the worst conditions. Collaborate with client to establish action plan. Steps (treatment) to reach client's clarified goals. Facilitate long range health planning and client action. Feedback on client actions and choices. Confrontation and challenging when necessary. Limitations of treatment. Solicit feedback on initial interview, co-diagnosis and long range planning and consultation appointment process.

Client Activities: Explores the best ways of achieving goals. Finds supportive resources to become healthy and change destructive habits (family, friends, support groups, information and classes.) Chooses action plan. Makes appointments.

Specifics: Treatment plan sheet, establish priorities of treatment, financial arrangements, mail long range plan to client.

This is a client-centered process and not a doctor-centered process. The client's right to make clarified health decisions is respected. We realize that in the absence of swelling, bleeding or pain, dentistry is discretionary. This enables the client to choose when he has dental work done by "making quality the constant and time the variable."

We respect the client's right to not have treatment done and try not to manipulate him to meet our values and needs. I realize this process flies in the face of what most doctors have been taught and believe—that one of their prime functions is to examine, diagnosis and to inform the patient of what needs to be done. Then they instruct the patient to schedule the appointments. If they do not, they are informed of the dire consequences of not having the treatment done. In the person-centered process, the assumption is that the client knows best. In a facilitative climate, the client will choose the best course of treatment and the optimum time to do the treatment.

The emergency or urgent client is treated differently. They are scheduled as quickly as possible to resolve the crisis. We don't offer lengthy sermons or explanations. We don't offer services that may in the end be harmful; for example, extracting a tooth when we can relieve the pain by extirpating the pulp. We do these services in an atmosphere of respect, comfort, caring and concern. After the crisis is past, we invite the person to return to discuss what happened and what can be done to prevent similar occurrences in the future.

The result of this way of bringing new people into our practice has been to enhance our relationships with our clients. It also enhances the type and quality of dentistry we do.

Health Therapies and Wellness Counseling

Commitments to helping a client learn, grow and heal have resulted in an emphasis on the importance of helping their client change destructive lifestyle habits and to become well. This is an evolution from the early days of preventive dentistry. Individual and group counseling is provided. The topics covered are: stress management, aerobic exercise programs, nutrition and weight control, money management, affirmations, guided imagery, relaxation exercises, referrals to appropriate community resources, lifework planning and health planning.

Besides dental services, person-centered practices have introduced several health therapies. Therapeutic touch, guided imagery, therapeutic massage, biofeedback, homeopathic treatment, acupuncture and a variety of other approaches. These practices have added these therapies, as they have found limitations in their traditional approach of dentistry and as their commitment to help their clients become healthier has grown.

Client Feedback

Does this approach work? The following letter from a client is an indication. "I just read your newsletter like a treasured letter from a close friend. I want to thank you for these monthly newsletters and for the caring atmosphere in your office. I recently came in for a cleaning and check up. I left the office feeling happy and loved, and it wasn't because I had no cavities! I, for one, appreciate the welcoming atmosphere in the office, the friendship and the feeling, insights, advice and hard work that goes into 'Adjuvant' (our newsletter). Thank you for being the special people you are."

"I am going to share this newsletter with my boss, who is seeking a new dentist for her daughter. It goes without saying, that I recommend Carlisle dentistry to all my friends. In an uncaring world, how refreshing to find an exception to the rule with you folks and good health and dental care to boot."

Yes, this approach does work. The evidence it works comes from responses like this letter and many other instances in the practices that have committed to this approach. Are there limitations to this approach? Yes there are.

Limitations of the Person-Centered Approach

Full application of this approach depends on the establishment of long term relationships. There are several instances where it is impossible or difficult to establish these relationships. In specialties where episodic care is the norm (oral surgery, endodontics), it is difficult to establish these relationships. However, dentists in these areas can still use the basics of the helping skills in their interactions with their patients.

The person-centered process is developmental and it takes time to implement. Some dentists give up before the benefits are evident.

Some dentists are not willing to pay the price to shift their values and beliefs to include the foundational beliefs of the person-centered approach.

It can result in reduced income initially as you go through the process of change.

There are patients who still want the doctor to be the boss and make all the decisions.

Clients have so much going on in their life, on an emotional level, that you cannot help them. They are unwilling to look at their emotional life and the impact it has on their health.

The threat of malpractice suits and the adversarial nature of some patients.

Some dentists feel this approach is too psychological, that being person-centered is too much like being a counselor. They would rather do the dentistry without interacting with the patient or getting into all that helping and wellness stuff.

Summary

The person-centered approach has been in dentistry since the middle sixties and it had developed and evolved over this time. Dentists have developed systems and nitty-gritty ways of using the approach in their practices. There are practical, effective ways of practicing that have produced results both in personal fulfillment, and in a financial return that is successful by any standards.

There is a price to be paid as the dentist and team make adjustments in their practices and belief systems. The process of change can be difficult, frustrating and rewarding. An understanding of the process of change is helpful in the personal and professional life of dentists and in understanding how clients change.

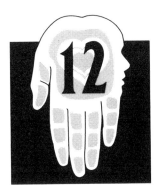

Change

Dentists are constantly involved with change in their own lives and in the lives of their clients. When clients come to see a dentist for the resolution of a problem, they are asking him for help in changing from a state of disease to a state of health or wellness. The facilitative conditions of a caring doctor-patient relationship help the client make needed changes in their lifestyle habits. For example, the resolution of a periodontal problem involves change in: the state of the periodontal sulcus from a toxic environment to a healthy environment, the change of destructive lifestyle habits, the creation of self-care strategies and the learning of new oral hygiene procedures.

In the dentist's life, he confronts changes in technology, changes in the attitudes and beliefs of his clients, changes in delivery systems and changes in the societal values and beliefs.

In the face of these challenges, it is important to understand the dynamics of change. We are experiencing more change than at any other time in the history of humankind. We are told that 25 per cent of all people who ever lived are living today; that 90 per cent of all scientists who ever lived are living now; the amount of technical information available doubles every seven years or less. E.A. Gutkind wrote in "Our World from the Air," "We are at one of the decisive turning points in the history of humanity, comparable to the domestication of animals, the invention of the earliest tools, the foundation of the first cities and the conception of the heliocentric universe." Change has always been a part of living. The difference we are experiencing now is the rapidity and depth of change. When we are in the midst of a change, it is difficult to have any sort of perspective. This results in a feeling of ignorance or ambiguity about change.

Elements of Change

What are the elements of change? What facilitates change and what detracts from change? A kaleidoscope serves as an apt metaphor for change. There are bits and pieces in our lives that are constantly rearranging themselves. They snap into focus with a startling clarity, only to blur and change again. I have moments of clarity and vision, only to have them disappear in a cloud of uncertainty. I try to grab the pieces that are changing, like feathers floating in the air, to arrest them in a fixed and immutable pattern. This process is futile, but I try anyway. My old ways of being keep rubbing against my new ways of being. The rubbing of old forms with new forms results in both being changed by the process.

Some definitions may help. Change is the process of movement from one place, thing, event, happening or state to another place, thing, event, happening or state. A change agent is a person who facilitates change or makes a difference in another person's life. In native cultures, the medicine men and women were seen as healing catalysts or change agents. I believe this is still true for modern day doctors.

There are two types of change. One is change from within—self-initiated change. The second is change from without—other-initiated change. The essential difference between self and other-directed change is choice. In self-initiated change, there is always choice. In other-initiated change, the person being changed does not have a choice. It comes from without and results in an automatic change in the person's life.

In health care, the distinction between self and other-directed change can be difficult. If a person has an automobile accident because of excessive alcohol consumption, is the accident self-initiated or other-initiated? Change in our life may be started by another person, but once the event has happened, we determine how we respond to change by the choices we make as to our response. This is what responsibility means, our ability to respond to what happens in our life.

If the person who caused the automobile accident was injured because of excessive alcohol consumption, then his injury was a result of self-initiated change. If the person who was injured was hit by a drunken driver, then his injuries were other-initiated. His response to the changes brought on by the accident will be self-initiated. Let's say he had maxillo-facial injuries because of the accident. The oral surgeon suggests physical therapy, nutritional supplements, self-care measures and oral hygiene procedures to facilitate the process of healing. The client needs to initiate changes in his personal habits to adapt to the suggestions of the oral surgeon. These changes are self-initiated.

In a person with periodontal disease, the person will face a series of decisions for self-initiated change in lifestyle habits to control periodontal disease. The need for the self-initiated change results from the lack of caring for his physical health.

Often major changes in a person's profession or culture will bring resistance to the perceived threat these changes will bring to a person's life. There will be an attempt to avoid or to stop these changes. What one person sees as a challenge, will be a quality of life threatening event to another.

The Semmelweiss Effect

Our culture views life as unchanging. When new ideas are introduced, there is usually resistance and denial to the new idea. The life of Ignaz Philiipp Semmelweiss, a Hungarian physician, illustrates this resistance to change. In 1846, when working at the Allgemeines Krankenhaus in Vienna, Semmelweiss noted that the maternal mortality in the ward attended by the medical students was far higher than that staffed by the nurses. Semmelweiss suspected the difference was due to the medical students coming to the maternity ward after their anatomy lab and infecting the parturient women. When he enforced the medical students washing their hands before examining the women, the maternal mortality rate fell dramatically. This discovery by Semmelweiss was fought, and he was persecuted by the prominent obstetricians of his time and he was forced to resign. He moved to Budapest where he became a professor of obstetrics in 1855.

In 1861, he published his great work on asepsis. The publication of this book initiated a new round of vilification of Semmelweiss. Semmelweiss did not live to see the general acceptance of his work, he suffered a mental breakdown and died in 1865 in an insane asylum. His courageous championship of asepsis ushered in a new era in medicine. Twenty-nine years later, a monument was built in honor of his discoveries in Budapest. Today, children learn at an early age to wash their hands before eating. The importance of cleanliness is a part of our culture now, a common ordinary fact we take for granted.

In retrospect, the attitude of the obstetricians of Semmelweiss's time seems ridiculous and archaic. This scenario repeats whenever new knowledge is introduced. The resistance to wellness, the philosophy of holistic health, changes in dental education and psychoneuroimmunology are current examples. The viewpoint that resulted in the denial of Semmelweiss' work says that as we discover truth and knowledge, there will be less knowledge that is unknown. There will be less need for change as more is known. A person believing in this viewpoint thinks that if only one more change is made, then everything will fall in place and no further changes will be made.

In my experience, life doesn't live this way. Change is integral to our lives, and it leads to an expansion of choices and options. Knowing more leads to knowing less. This is a paradox, the more we learn, the more we realize that there are more things that we do not know or are mysteries in our life than what we know. This leads to the need to become comfortable with ambiguity and trusting in the process of change instead of believing that we can control life and change.

Prigogine's Theory of Dissapative Structures

Ilya Prigogine's theory of dissapative structures supports this view. Prigogine, a physical chemist from Belgium, won the 1977 Nobel Prize in chemistry for his theory of dissapative structures. In his book, *From Being To Becoming*, he states, "The increased limitation of deterministic laws means that we go from a universe that is closed, in which all is given, to a new one that is open to fluctuations, to innovation." As a person or society experiences more complexity, it is more susceptible to change, to "perturbations." Change is not a smoothly ascending linear process, but is a process of seemingly random bursts that lead to jumps or paradigm shifts in knowledge. "There are always fluctuations, instabilities to drive the system into new dimensions."

The clash of these two world views (an open universe as opposed to a closed universe) increases the anxiety in our society. This clash results in dissonance in people's life. Stress results and some people are challenged by the dissonance and others are threatened. In our dental practice, some of our patients grow and change because of these challenges, and others become ill because of the perceived threat.

Observations on Change

The following observations have helped me understand the process of change:

✦ Risk is always involved in change.
✦ The potential of loss or gain is involved in change.
✦ Stress is involved in change.
✦ Change can be good or bad.
✦ All change involves learning, and all learning involves change.
✦ The closer something is to you the harder it is to change.
✦ The longer something has been done, the harder it is to change.
✦ Change is an on going process.
✦ Fundamental change is harder than superficial change.
✦ Change is holistic-it effects all parts of your life.
✦ Change can be simple or complex-gradual or instantaneous.
✦ The frequency, duration and depth of change determines how stressful it is.

Each time there is change, energy is released and we have the potential to use that energy synergistically or destructively. It is our perception of how change effects our life that determines its impact.

I have served on the local board of directors of Hospice. The nurses and volunteers who work with terminally ill people report that some of their clients transform their lives because of their illness. They report that the client's healing comes from a healing of the client's attitudes and beliefs. They say that these clients who experience attitudinal healing are the most joyous and serene people they know. What is perceived as the most traumatic event in a person's life has been changed into a transformational spiritual experience by these people.

What are some models of change?

Three Models of Change

The following models have helped me to understand the process of change. In the first Dr. Becoming letter, I discussed Keleman's model of change.

Endings → Beginnings → Middle Ground → New Forms

Figure 4.

To review, Keleman said that to have beginnings, we first need to have endings. We have to decide to stop an activity or behavior. In dieting, a person needs to decide to stop overeating. Then he begins new behavior, a new way of eating. This new behavior propels him into the middle ground, which is a time of going back and forth between the new behavior, that Keleman called new forms, and the old patterns or forms. Over time, when the intent to change is strong enough, the new forms gradually replace the old forms and new habits form.

People often crash on the rocks of the discomfort of the new forms. An unknown author described this phenomenon this way.

Awareness → uninformed optimism → informed pessimism →

hopeful realism → informed optimism → enlightenment

Figure 5.

As a person becomes *aware* of the need to make some changes in his life, he becomes excited about these changes and has an *uninformed optimism* of the good things that will come about. Then if things don't work out the way he planned, he is crushed and sees all the reasons his idea won't work. This leads to *informed pessimism*. This stage is a critical one and most people give up at this point instead of understanding that this stage provides an opportunity to learn from their mistakes. They are trapped in a cycle of being excited about an idea, trying it out, being disappointed in the results and giving up. Those who work through the disappointment of informed pessimism see a way that the idea can work. They learn from the disappointment and experience *hopeful realism*. They realistically see how their idea can work out. They try the revised idea and experience success. This success leads to *informed opti- mism*. If they integrate the new learning into the rest of their life, they experience a paradigm shift and become *enlightened* and whole.

The model of transformational change that I have developed looks like this:

Unawareness → Awareness → Ah-ha! → Born Again → Integration → Transcendence.

Figure 6.

Most of us are *unaware* of the need to change until an event happens in our life. This event leads to the glimmer of *awareness*. The glimmer may stay just an awareness or an *Ah-ha!* may occur and you see the world in a new way; you feel your life transform with born again fervor. In the born again *phase* you experience the arrogance of newness. You immediately assume that you have made the great leap and have knowledge that no one else has. You feel that others are not as enlightened as you are, and your mission in life is to help them see the world as you see it. The born again phase can be a very obnoxious phase to those around you as their integrity detectors ring like a fire alarm, but it is necessary because there is tremendous energy created in this phase. The energy is vitally necessary to help the person move through all of the incongruities that he discovers in his life. The born again one does not live his life like he proselytizes to others to live their life. This energy enables him to work through and learn from these incongruities, and to begin integrating this new way of being into his life in a way that he becomes more congruent. After *integration*, he may help others by the congruence of his actions. As a person integrates these insights into his life, he feels a feeling of *transcendence*, of seeing life as a spiritual journey, as going beyond the ego and seeing how he is connected to everything and everyone in the universe.

Understanding Change

Understanding change comes from looking back and seeing how the process of change can be trusted. But life seems so confusing and ambiguous in the moment of change. It may seem in the moment of change that the change could not possibly turn out well. Soren Kierkegard said it best, "Life is best understood backwards, but must be lived forwards." Change involves giving something up; the death of an idea, a relationship, a dream, a person, a way of eating, a technique, a substance. Change can set up a process of grieving the loss of the old, and one can move through the stages of grief-denial, anger, acceptance. What we are giving up may be abusive to our health or to our very being. At least we know what it is. It is the unknown about change that is so threatening to many people. The threat of change is also perceptual. What is threatening to one person is no big deal to another. It is the perception of the threat of change, instead of the perception of challenge, which often stops people from changing.

Obviously there are different levels of change that can range from the cataclysmic (divorce, life threatening disease, loss of a job) to daily changes (a change in a schedule, exercise routines, and time of day when you eat).

Resistors to Change

Here are some things that make change difficult: rigidity in systems or ideas, educational and family systems that punish mistakes, an emphasis on being right, an emphasis on playing it safe, fear of loss, fear of failure, the length of time the old habit has been in existence and past failures in making changes.

A person who has not been successful in making changes in his life will be more reluctant to initiate further changes. His experience with change has not been good. Failure in change has created raw, tender spots in the person's being. When change is perceived as threatening to these tender spots, the person closes like a turtle to protect these vulnerable areas. They associate feelings of failure, diminished self esteem and reduced self-worth with change.

Mistakes As Agents of Change

When we make mistakes, we never learn less. Somehow our culture and thinking lead to the feeling that we should not make mistakes and we punish people for making mistakes. We are trained to not make mistakes. Buckminster Fuller's quote in *Critical Path*, applies again, "It is only at the moment of humans' realistic admission to selves of having made a mistake that they are closest to that mysterious integrity governing the universe. — The courage to adhere to the truth as we learn it involves then, the courage to face ourselves with the clear admission of all the mistakes we have made. Mistakes are sins only when not admitted. Etymologically, sin means omission where admission should have occurred."

Facilitating Change

The person-centered approach helps to facilitate the process of change by helping dentists and clients open and move. The process of change places a premium on creating a growth promoting climate for dentists and their clients as they move through the change process. Carl Rogers said that "self acceptance is the beginning of change." This acceptance of where one is—good or bad—leads to change. (Even surrender or resignation to where one is can lead to change) The greater a feeling of self-worth and self-esteem a person has, the easier it is for them to change. A person's feeling of self worth is increased by another's unconditional acceptance and understanding of them.

Past successes at change help increase a person's courage and confidence to initiate further changes in their life. A client who has made successful changes in his life will be more open to further changes, than one who has not been successful in making changes. I have found that a person who is already exercising, who has learned to manage his stress or has lost weight, will be more open to suggestions to change. They have learned the benefits of change and have come to thrive on change and may even seek out areas to change in their life. They have learned that successful change increases their feeling of self worth and self esteem. Their self-confidence has been enhanced, and they are more willing to risk. They live more in the moment and do not fear the future or dwell on past mistakes. They can positively create an image of themselves making the change.

Changing Health Habits

Health habits are among the most difficult to change. It seems that a quality of life threatening condition needs to occur or change needs to be piggybacked on other successful change as was discussed above. Health habits are close to a person's core of being. These health habits often fill voids in their lives and serve as crutches to prop up a person's life. Change in these habits is often viewed as threatening to clients. Helping clients to imagine how the change will enhance their feeling of well being, self-esteem and self-worth, are the beginning points of change. These appeals can be in terms of Roy Garn's emotional appeals of self-preservation, money, recognition or romance. The change will help them preserve or achieve health or well being, to be comfortable, save money, be more attractive, to attract attention and feel more powerful.

Another deterrent to change for some people is the amount of change in their life. There may be so much going on in their lives that the thought of one more thing to change is too overwhelming. This is the "Stop the World, I want to Get Off" syndrome. A client came to see me for the recementation of a crown that was loose. The tooth was badly decayed and needed to be removed. A glance at the rest of his mouth told me he was in trouble. He had periodontal disease, and several of his other teeth were in need of restoration. The correction of these problems would be expensive.

I asked him about his life, where he worked, and when he had moved to Ft.Collins. He said that he had recently been transferred by his company to Ft. Collins. It was a very stressful time for him. He had recently been divorced. He had not wanted to move to Ft. Collins, but his company had left him no choice. It was move or lose his job. His family was still back in the Midwest. He was responsible for the educational expenses of his two children in college. He was paying alimony. A new granddaughter had recently been born and he had not been back to see her. He had started a relationship with a woman, in his former town, just before his move to Colorado, and she had just moved to Florida. He wanted to see her. He wanted to find a job and move back to his old town.

I listened to him, and replied; "It seems to me that there is a lot of stress going on in your life. You feel financial and emotional demands from all sides. I feel a dilemma, because I see trouble for you dentally. You have some things going on that if they are not taken care of may result in the loss of some teeth. It will be expensive to treat these conditions, and this is the last thing you want at this time."

He said, "You're right, is there anything we can do to take care of the immediate problems? I would rather have the teeth pulled than put any major amount of money in them now." Having the dental work could be the straw that broke his back, so we worked out a holding treatment that would keep his dental condition from deteriorating. We tried to not make many demands dentally. We postponed the major treatment until a time when his life was calmer and he could afford it.

People do want to change, grow and become more fully integrated persons. They want to achieve health and well being; to become whole. Circumstances and events in people lives often seem to blur this drive much as the static on the radio interferes with the clear reception of a radio signal. In the example above, the person was moving toward health in his own way. My values as a dentist led me to feel that his dental health was a high priority. His values of getting his life in balance led him to place higher priorities on the other areas of his life- like alimony, tuition, return to his hometown, seeing his girlfriend—than on his dental needs. I tried to do the minimum amount of dentistry that would get him through this time of change and still enable him to have the major work done later without endangering his health.

Precessional Effects—An Example

Buckminster Fuller wrote about the precessional effect. He said it is often the events that happen along the way toward a goal that are most important. The goal provides us the direction to move in, but it is what happens, often at 90 degrees, which provides the most growth and change in our lives.

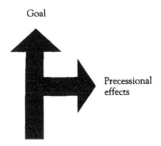

Figure 7. Buckminster Fuller's Precessional Effect

In the mid 1980's, I experienced a growing sense of dissatisfaction with my practice of dentistry. I felt like I was not receiving what I was putting into my practice. My clients were not appreciating all the changes I had made and were not interested in wellness and the ways in which we helped. I started considering my options: selling my practice and becoming a wellness consultant, moving to another city and starting a new dental practice, teaching in dental school, doing research or specialty training, consulting and lecturing in dentistry.

I entered career counseling to see what insight counseling would give me. It was an agonizing time for me because I had lost the vision and meaning of my life's work. I had burnt out. Eventually, with my wife's support, I decided to sell my practice and take a sabbatical. I would travel for a year to let the answer come to me instead of figuring out the next step. I put my practice up for sale and informed my clients by letter of my decision to leave. This is the letter that I sent.

I began the letter with a quotation from Richard Bach's *Illusions* about a village of creatures that lived along the bottom of a river. Bach talked about the creatures clinging tightly to the rocks and twigs on the river bottom. One of the creatures decided to let go and trust that the current knew where it was going. The other creatures laughed at him and called him a fool. The creature let go and was buffeted and crashed on the rocks. He refused to cling to the rocks and was carried on the current and was no longer bruised and buffeted. Bach wrote, "The river delights to lift us free, if we only dare to let go. Our work is this voyage, this adventure."

I then wrote:

> "This quotation is from the beginning of Richard Bach's book Illusions. *I received it as part of a brochure announcing a workshop. I did not attend the workshop, but I did reread* Illusions. *The quotation came at the right time for me and it affirmed a decision Kirsten and I had just made. The decision was to transfer our dental practice to another dentist and take a year's sabbatical and let the current carry us to the next part of our life."*

> "Kirsten and I had been considering this decision for the past year. It was an agonizing time for us, as we vacillated between starting the next step or staying. When we made the decision to take sometime to let the next step emerge, we finally decided to let go of our dental practice."

"There are many aspects to this decision. Some of them are: I have been practicing dentistry for 24 years, I am 45 years old, I have reached and exceeded many of the goals I had set for myself and I have not reached others, I have had other interests emerge about wellness and whole person approaches. The spiritual part of my life has become increasingly important. The most significant part is—It is time for a change."

"When will this change occur? Probably late this year or early next year. Our dental practice will remain fully functioning and available to take care of your dental needs during and after this transition period. *We are currently looking for a dentist that we feel will be technically, personally and philosophically compatible with us and you to assume our practice. It is very important to us to have a good transition of our practice with you."*

"The hardest part of our decision was leaving you and the other people in our practice. We have come to value you as both clients and friends, and we will deeply miss our contact with you. From a personal and professional standpoint, I have learned a tremendous amount because of my practice of dentistry with you. I thank you for your caring, concern and support over the past 18 years."

"With sincere gratitude,

Lynn D. Carlisle, D.D.S."

I was going to make a major change in my life. (This whole year was filled with many sleepless nights as I vacillated between the excitement and fear of the change I had decided to make in my life. It was one of the hardest years in my life.) For one year, I was unable to sell my practice. I finally had a buyer for my dental equipment, another buyer for my house, and a buyer for my client's records. It was very complex, but I had decided to go for it and a date was set to sign a letter of intent to sell the equipment. The night before I was to sign the letter of intent was a sleepless one, as I wrestled with my decision to leave dentistry. Something happened during the night. The next morning, I told my wife that I decided to stay. She thought I was crazy because the day before I was excited about selling and beginning our sabbatical. I sent another letter to my clients telling them of my decision to stay.

We Are Staying

"*I had decided to take the years' sabbatical to find out what I wanted to do with the next part of my life and it turned out to be what I have been doing—practicing dentistry and living in Fort Collins.*"

"*How I arrived at the decision to stay is a long story. The essence is that I went on the journey I wanted to go on without taking an external trip. But, boy did I take an internal one! I 'tumbled and smashed across a lot of rocks' as I wrestled with my decision to sell my practice.*"

"*When I had an offer to buy my practice, I panicked and spent a heart wrenching month struggling with my decision to sell. The morning before I was scheduled to sign the letter of intent, I decided to stay. Talk about brinkmanship. The decision to stay has relieved my anxiety and I am excited about practicing dentistry again.*"

"*What I have been experiencing the last 2–3 years was probably a combination of burn out and mid-career crises. What I had thought was external—dentistry, Fort Collins, wanting to do other things—turned out to be internal and the way I was seeing things. So my voyage of discovery was not in seeking new vistas—but in having new eyes.*"

"*When I decided to stay, those externals changed. I realized how much I valued our clients, my friends, my dental lab, Fort Collins, the mountains, my house, my office, my co-workers and my profession. What I was looking for was already here.*"

"*So, I am staying—in the same profession, same office, same city, same house, (with the same patient wife). The current lifted me free and my adventure brought me home. I find it difficult to tell you how the past year has changed the way I view my work—but I will try. It has changed from a way of making a living to a way of expressing the way I live. I am excited about dentistry and Fort Collins, and feel like I am beginning again.*"

"*I am looking forward to seeing you and giving you the nitty-gritty. Also, I would like to ask you for your help in my beginning again by referring your friends, neighbors, family and colleagues to us. I need your help in building my practice again.*"

*"Thank you for your understanding and support of me as
I went through my journey."*

Warmly,

Lynn

I had sought peace and wholeness by my decision to leave
dentistry. Surprisingly, to me and my wife, this decision had resulted precessionally in a deepening of meaning and commitment to
dentistry. In an inscription to me in her book, *The Human Patient*,
Naomi Remen had written "Dear Lynn—The voyage of discovery
lies not in seeking new vistas, but in having new eyes—I wish you
continuing joy in your work." I had opened her book up four years
later to the day that she had written this inscription to me. I learned
the greater meaning of my practice of dentistry and learned to trust
that changes that seem to be the most traumatic are often the greatest
learning experiences and are the most enriching.

Campbell's Hero's Journey

The result of change can be exhilarating or discouraging.

Often, when a person is in the midst of change, all he can see is
the chaos that changes create. The models of change used in this
chapter all include going from the known to the unknown. They
include: a middle ground, a time of doubt and pessimism, a time of
trials, a time of integration in which chaos, fear, disappointment and
anxiety occur.

Joseph Campbell, a mythologist, has written about the process
of change in *The Hero with a Thousand Faces*. Campbell uses the
myths from different cultures to show how these cultures understood
and coped with change. Campbell defines a hero as "someone (male
or female) who has given his or her life to something bigger than
oneself." He says that there are two deeds—one is physical and the
other is spiritual. In both deeds, the person experiences a series of
adventures beyond the ordinary, to discover what has been lost or
to discover something new. The adventure is a process of transformation—a going and a returning.

The hero's journey is a time of trials in which the person's
mettle is tested to see if he has the courage, the knowledge and the

capacity to serve. The hero loses himself to some higher end or to another person. In this vision quest what is missing in the hero's life is discovered. The challenge to the hero is to stay with the discovery of the vision quest—what he calls a boon—and bring it back into his ordinary world. Campbell acknowledges the difficulty of doing this. He also talks about the hero's journey as it relates to self-initiated change and other-initiated change. Campbell feels it is the person's courage in responding to the self or other-initiated change that determines if he is worthy of being called a hero.

It is important that wisdom and common sense be used as the hero follows the path of his desire, enthusiasm and emotion. He uses the example of Daedalus, who made wings for himself and his son Icarus to use to fly. Daedalus gave his son the advice to "Fly the middle way. Don't fly too high, or the sun will melt the wax on your wings, and you will fall. Don't fly too low, or the tides of the sea will catch you." Daedalus heeded his own advice and flew the middle way and his son became ecstatic and flew too high and fell into the sea.

The trials may result in suffering and in the myths of being crucified, but out of the suffering and endings come beginnings and new life. Campbell felt it is important to follow the hints that come from the mythological journey, to find a guru -a teacher who helps the prospective hero bring his own energies into play, or a book that speaks to one personally about the trials they are experiencing.

Campbell felt myths inspire the possibility of realizing your perfection, of finding the strength to bring you the "soul's high adventure," which is to find your bliss and then to "Follow your bliss." This is Campbell's famous phrase to find a life's work that you enjoy and to follow it as it creates the soul's high adventure. This adventure leads one to discover that each person is a unique creature and their gift to the world will come out of the fulfillment of each person's potentialities and not those of another. From this adventure, the hero finds what makes a person happy and to stay with it no matter what others say. This is following your bliss and when a person's bliss is followed, he finds it within himself. Campbell says that this is the adventure that change initiates and it is "the adventure of being alive."

Summary

Through this adventure, the hero becomes the master of change instead of the victim or recipient of change. Instead of being an end or a threat to a person's life, change can lead to the transformation of a person's life. An appreciation and understanding of the purpose and potential of change can lead the dentist and client to learning, growth and change. The "hero's journey" involves trials and tribulations—a wounding of the dentist in his role as a healer that leads to the potential for healing in the client and dentist.

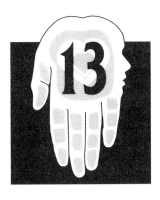

The Wounded Healer

The idea of the wounded healer has run, like a current through the history of health and healing. In ancient times, the predecessors of modern doctors were shamans, witch doctors, priests and medicine men and women. These ancient doctors often became a "healer" because of a personal experience with a physical, emotional or spiritual illness or disease. If they did not have a personal transformative experience, they went through rites of initiation that gave them an experience of their inner world and how it influenced their outer world. Their life experience in combination with their skills as a doctor, counselor, teacher and priest helped them in their roles as facilitators of healing.

Origins of the Wounded Healer

The Greek mythological figure Chiron, is often called the origin of the idea of the wounded healer. According to this myth, during a battle Chiron was wounded in the knee with a poisoned arrow. The wound was incurable, but because Chiron was immortal he could not die, nor could he be cured. Chiron, who was a centaur—half man and half horse—became the greatest teacher of medicine of his time because of his wound. He taught many early Greek physicians. Among them was Asclepius, who, in Greek mythology is regarded as the father of healing and medicine. A central teaching, which Chiron passed onto Asclepius, was the wisdom available to him through acknowledging his woundedness.

A central theme in Jean Auel's book *Clan of the Cave Bear*, is the relationship between the crippled Shaman, Creb, and the heroine, Ayla. Because of their disabilities, both in their own way were outcasts. Creb's disability was his physical deformities and Ayla's was her heritage; she was not of the Clan but of the Others, a different race. Their experiences of these disabilities led to their effectiveness as the healers of the Clan.

Wounded healers still exist today within each of us. This idea has been forced underground because of the myth of perfection, of omnipotence, of being the all-knowing and all-powerful one, which we have taken on like an ill-fitting cloak. We do not acknowledge our woundedness—our feelings of failure when a procedure does not go well, our feelings of not doing enough when we are unable to figuratively or literally save the life of a person, the feeling of loneliness and isolation in our work with our patients and feelings that no one else has the doubts and problems we have.

Paradoxically, these experiences and feelings are the ones that enable us to be more effective doctors as we enter the lives of our clients and understand their fear and anxiety because we have experienced similar fears and anxieties in our own lives. Our feelings of fear and failure often provide us with the greatest opportunities for learning, growth, and change as we struggle to make sense out of what on the surface seems senseless. Larry Dossey, M.D., in *Beyond Illness*, writes "The greatest healers, however, do not participate in this myth of perfection. They sense their own limitations as surely as they know their strengths. They know the necessity of illness in human life and its dynamic interrelatedness with health. For them the light and shadows are both essential ingredients of healthiness, and they do not attempt to ignore one in favor of the other." (Dossey 1985, p. 195–6).

Vale of Tears

Most effective doctors have gone through a vale of tears, a time of trial and tribulation, in their personal or practice life. This vale of tears has transformed their world view, their vision of what doctoring means to them. L.D. Pankey talks about how his mother's premature loss of her teeth at an early age of 42, led to his commitment to devote his dental career to saving teeth. "It was a letter from my mother who said, 'I am happy you are doing well in your practice, but I hope you are not doing to your patients what has been done to me. I have had all my teeth out and now have dentures. This has been the unhappiest experience of my life'." Pankey said in relating how he felt that "The shock of it all and the considerable thought I gave it opened the door to a vision that the dentist's responsibility and goal should be to save patients' teeth for a lifetime, if at all possible." The experience of his mother and his own experience of doing similar treatments "to other people's mothers, what another dentist had done to mine sickened me." It led to his decision, "I would never take out another tooth as long as I lived." (A Philosophy of the Practice of Dentistry, Pankey, Davis, 1985). In a lecture he gave sixty years later, his voice still quivered with emotion, as he described his feelings at the time he received his mother's letter.

Bob Barkley described a similar feeling of failure at his inability to help one of his favorite high school cheerleaders save her teeth. "Extremely anxious to help, I assured her that if she improved her brushing we could do wonders. Then I prescribed only such repair work as seemed absolutely necessary. Even these holding action estimates seemed monumental to a young family with four small children. The next time I saw her I could have cried—she had committed dental suicide in another dental office and was waiting for her gums to heal before getting dentures. 'Never again' I told myself, 'will I offer a patient something he cannot accept, nor will I allow my holding action to cost more than tooth removal and dentures. In my office, it will be cheaper to keep teeth than to lose them. I will make prevention pay off.'" *(Barkley, 1972) Both Pankey and Barkley's woundedness led to a series of events that transformed their lives and changed the practice of dentistry.*

My own experience of wounding came as a result of a series of events that included a divorce, a malpractice suit, the "Semmelweiss" effect of being one of the first people to introduce holistic health and wellness in my city and my decision to sell my practice and later my decision to stay in practice.

For other dentists, their experience of wounding came from the loss of key team members, mistakes in treatment or diagnosis, failed restorations, bad results, disgruntled patients, malpractice suits, financial difficulties and the myriad of other instances of wounding that are part of a dental practice.

The central theme in all these people's experiences was a deep dissatisfaction, a feeling of being incompetent, of having failed—of being wounded—that led to a transformative experience that gave a greater vision, a sense of new meaning and purpose to their professional lives. The deep dissatisfaction and feelings of failure led them to the hero's journey.

Pain and Suffering

Doctoring involves pain and suffering, both our clients and our own. In our professional life, we work with people who are in pain and are suffering. Usually, when our clients are experiencing pain and suffering, they are not fully themselves. Often, the fear and anxiety (fear results from that which is known, anxiety results from that which is unknown) that pain and suffering cause can make the patient childlike and sometimes crazy (they are not in touch with what is going on within themselves). This fear and anxiety manifests in anger, crying, whining, cancellations, postponing treatment, endless questions, vindictiveness, lawsuits, denial and many other manifestations of human emotions. This pain and suffering includes the overt or covert patient hostility referred to in chapters four and eight that dentists are exposed to. Cathy Kamensky, Laura Museo and Sandra Naiman wrote an article titled "Who's Killing the American Dentist," concerning this patient hostility. They felt patient hostility resulted from the lack of control the patient has when dental work is done and "it is a deeply somatic response to the violation of a private space." In their words, the dentist gets emotionally "zapped" by the patient's hostility.

Sometimes, in our treatment and interactions with patients, there is just pain and suffering and life does not make sense. Doctors feel impotent because they do not understand why so much pain and suffering occurs in people's lives, including their own.

We have been taught largely through modeling experiences to wall ourselves off from this pain and suffering. We distance ourselves at a time when our human presence is most needed by our clients. We use these same defense mechanisms with our own pain and suffering. It fails miserably as the statistics on divorce, depression, drug and alcohol abuse, failed partnerships and burn out in doctors illustrate.

I believe the block to experiencing our fears and our pain and suffering is that these fears will get stuck and we will be unable to rid ourselves of them. It is another paradox, that to go through pain and suffering, we must acknowledge and express the presence of pain and suffering in our lives; to be open to it and allow it to flow through without trying to justify our fear and anxiety or blame others. We must confront and wrestle with our own pain and suffering before we can help others with their pain and suffering.

Psychologically healthy people are in touch with their feelings and can fully express these feelings. This expression helps the feelings to flow through and not get stuck. In Modern Man in Search of a Soul, Carl Jung wrote:

> "No one pays the doctor for his introspective efforts: and moreover, we are generally not interested enough in ourselves. Again, we so commonly undervalue the deeper aspects of the human psyche that we hold self-examination or preoccupation with ourselves to be almost morbid. We evidently suspect ourselves of harboring rather unwholesome things all too reminiscent of a sickroom. The physician must overcome these resistances in himself, for who can educate others while he remains uneducated? Who can enlighten his fellows while still in the dark about himself, and who can purify if he is himself unclean?"

Bernie Seigel, M.D. wrote of his experience in how "This expanded outlook helps a doctor to inspire hope, give with the heart as well as the head and hands, keep ego in the background and share major decisions with the patient. Such an approach rewards the physician as well as the patient. The love returns in words and looks of gratitude, in cards, and letters and in little gifts for the office, all of which restore you. A doctor who acts out of love doesn't burn out. He or she may be tired physically, but not emotionally."

Becoming a Warrior

My vision of a person-centered doctor as a warrior is one of a doctor who experiences the sadness, fear and hurt from his mistakes, his inability to help and cure all of his patients. He feels the frustration of not being understood by his patients, colleagues and co-workers. In this sadness, fear and hurt, he is brave and fearless enough to still reach out and touch the ground of goodness he believes exists in human beings. This process awakens his "sad and tender heart" and allows him to share this heart with others. By acknowledging his woundedness, he brings light into the darkness generated by his fear and anxieties. His fears become unstuck instead of stuck.

Working with our own and other's pain and suffering requires an understanding of the tradition of human warriorship that is founded upon the belief that "there is a basic human wisdom that can help to solve our world's problems." This tradition has existed in many cultures at many times in our history: Native American Indian, Tibetan Shambhala teachings, Japanese samuri tradition, the Christian and Jewish traditions of which King Arthur and King David are examples.

Chogyam Trungpa, a Buddhist meditation master, scholar and artist, gave the following explanation of the Shambhala vision of warriorship:

> "Warriorship in this context is the tradition of human bravery, or the tradition of fearlessness. — The key to warrior-ship—is not being afraid of who you are. — In the face of the world's great problems, we can be heroic and kind at the same time. — There is something basically good about our existence as human beings. Unless we can discover that ground of good-ness in our own lives, we cannot hope to improve the lives of others. — The essence of warriorship, or the essence of brav-ery, is refusing to give up on anyone or anything."
> (Shambhala—The Sacred Path of the Warrior. 1984).

In this kind of warriorship, when you appreciate yourself, your mind and body, "you begin to contact the fundamental notion of basic goodness in yourself. Developing tenderness toward yourself allows you to see both your problems and your potential accurately." This kind of gentleness toward yourself and appreciation of yourself provides the ground for helping yourself and others. So, in the Shambhala vision of warriorship, one who is a warrior is brave and fearless because he has discovered the touchstone of his own basic goodness, and in touching his own goodness is able to perceive similar goodness in others. The gentle warrior has learned how to help and heal from going through the vale of tears his woundedness created. This leads him to develop tenderness, caring, compassion, gentleness and appreciation for himself and others.

Reaching Out

If you experience your woundedness in isolation, without the help of others, your chance of healing yourself and helping others is problematical. The expression of my own woundedness is helped greatly by the presence of supportive people and groups in my life. There are five groups that provide me with precious support when I reach out to them (and when I do not).

One is a group that includes my wife, family and friends outside of dentistry. They are my companions on my life's journey and are able to help, love and support me when I am wounded. They are also wonderful playmates to take me into the world of re-creation. Being with them provides this outlet of freedom.

Second are my co-workers, the people I work with on a daily basis. I am most influenced by these people, because they are most available to me. They often can sense when something is going on with me before I am consciously aware of it. If I am disturbed by a patient or by a mistake I have made, they are wonderful listeners when I express my feelings of frustration, hurt or anger. A hug, an understanding glance, from them helps me to know I am understood. This was not true early in my career, but as I became more understanding, respectful, and empathic toward my co-workers, they mirrored these attitudes to me.

The third group is my clients. I find that as I have expressed my humanness and vulnerability, they have responded with support and compassion. Through my practice newsletter, our client advisory board, and my one to one interaction with my clients, I have increasingly shared more of myself with results that have startled me. My client's gratitude and support have been one of the most serendipitous experiences of my life. Initially, I thought I was sharing for my client's benefit, that I was being a good helper by being genuine and congruent. This did help my clients, and they began expressing their concern, their gratitude and appreciation for me. In helping them, in caring for them, they reciprocally did the same for me.

The fourth is a study group of fellow dentists. I helped organize this group in 1977. Our initial focus was on technical aspects of dentistry, particularly restorative dentistry, and occlusal/muscle/temporomandibular joint dysfunction. Gradually, as we came to trust each other, we began to discuss our feelings about our personal and professional lives. We discussed our hurts and frustrations with cases that had failed; our exasperation in carrying out changes in our practices, our financial problems, the clients and staff with whom we were frustrated. We asked each others advice on cases, on how to work with difficult staff or client problems. We talked of our personal lives. During our time together, there have been divorces, marital problems, bankruptcies, heart attacks, burn out, problems with children, law suits, poor investments, and unfulfilled hopes, dreams and visions. There have also been moments of joy and achievement as we attained financial goals and honors, as children married, as articles were published, as opportunities to give back to dentistry arose and there was recognition of the members' achievement of technical excellence in the practice of dentistry. We became friends, counselors and teachers to each other. We came to love each other.

In some unique ways, this group and the fifth group listed below, are the most valuable to me. They are the most valuable, because they alone have the depth of understanding about me as a dentist because they are fellow dentists. Only they have experienced what it is like to be a dentist with the attendant highs and lows. They have the wealth of their life's experience as a dentist to draw upon to understand my trials and tribulations as a dentist. As we came to trust, care and love each other, this common bond helped us to enter each other's world and express a deep empathic understanding of what it was like to be a dentist.

The fifth group is an extended family of dental professionals in the U.S. and Canada. I have met these people because of my attendance and facilitation of workshops, exploring the dimensions of the person-centered approach in dentistry. It has been invaluable to me to interact with fellow travelers and to share common hopes and frustrations with the path we have chosen.

Who Will Heal the Healers?

Cecil E. Burney, Jr., a Jungian psychotherapist, captured the essence of this collegial bond beautifully in his poem, "The Legacy after the Fact."

> Who will heal the healers
> If not the healers themselves?
> Knowing each other
> Trusting each other
> Touching each other
> Finding each other again and again
>   with tenderness.

> Who will heal the healers
> If not the healers themselves?
> Putting aside the demands of profession
> And healing each other not with power
>   but with love.
> Who will heal the healers

If not the healers themselves?
Music itself is healing for them.
Lame Chiron taught Asklepious to heal
but he also taught music:
"He educated them to be physicians
    and turned their minds to music
And made them into just men."*

Who will heal us
If we do not heal each other?
With love
And with companionship
And with empathy
And with joy.

We enter the play of our life together
    And become whole
Singing and playing and loving and healing.

There is justice for us where we venture to go.

*Philostratus, *Heroicus*

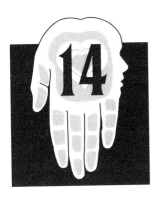

Take Care of Yourself, Doc

"Take care of yourself, doc!" A client once said that to me when I told him I was going through a tough time in my life. This is excellent advice. The saying that you can't give from empty pockets is very appropriate for dentists. The emphasis of dental school, continuing education seminars, articles and books is on what the dentist needs to do to provide care for his clients. In the dentist's role as a caregiver, there is the potential for the dentist to focus on giving his best care, skill and judgement to his clients and patients. The danger for the dentist is that he does not also give to himself. When one feels wounded one needs to take time to heal.

Care For the Caregiver

At its highest and best, caregiving includes the giver of care, here the dentist, giving to himself and giving to his client. The statistics on stress, burnout, addictions and career dissatisfaction in dentists, poignantly show that this reciprocal giving to the client and himself is often absent in dentists. There is a danger in writing a book on helping that an implied message is that helping and caregiving is a one way process from the dentist to his client. I don't feel that this is true. I feel the dentist needs to give to himself in direct proportion to the care he gives his client.

Dentistry often is hard work and is the source of distress for the dentist. A myriad of factors lead to distress: the rapidity of change in the dentists and clients lives, economic stresses, mistakes, the threat of malpractice suits, unrealistic client or patient expectations, dissatisfied clients or patients, staff or team problems, practice management problems, cash flow problems, financial difficulties, unrealistic expectations by the dentist, the perfectionistic and reductionistic residue of dentist's training, third party encroachments in dentistry, the "busyness" problem, feelings of not doing or being enough, worrying, fear, anxiety etc. The list often seems endless.

There is a tendency to think, as I wrote in the first Dr. Becoming letter, that if only I find the magic ingredient(s), then all my problems will be solved and there would be no stress in my life. This is an unrealistic expectation. Life is a collage of hopes, fears, joys, problems and frustrations. This life cannot be avoided. The challenge is how do we respond to the hopes, fears, joys, problems and frustrations in our lives. How do we care for ourselves as we respond to these challenges?

The challenge of responding to the fears, frustrations and problems in our lives is enough to make all of us Buddhists, to view all of the happenings in our lives as just "grist for our mills"; to view these happenings with interest and curiosity but without attachment, without getting bound up in the "What ifs?," "Ain't it awfuls" and other thoughts that usually accompany the negative happenings in our lives. This would be a significant accomplishment and it is one I aspire to, but I haven't achieved it yet. At this time, my life goal is to get the butterflies in my stomach to fly in formation, as Rob Gilbert said in his quotation, "It's all right to have butterflies in your stomach. Just get them to fly in formation."

I am intimidated by writing about caring for the caregiver. I am concerned that I will preach and act like I have solved all of my life's problems, or I will be a cheerleader and say if only you think positively everything will be O.K. I haven't solved all my problems and I will probably do a little cheerleading. This is probably why I aspire to getting my butterflies to fly in formation.

Quotes

Truckloads of books have been written on what to do to change parts of people's lives that they don't like. Often these books both help and hinder one in his quest for happiness. This is probably due to the paradoxical nature of life. I am a collector of quotes and would like to share the following quotes with you. There will be a paradoxical nature between some quotes. Life is often paradoxical.

"Courage is doing what you're afraid to do. There can be no courage unless you're scared." (Eddie Rickenbacker)

"When you make a mistake, admit it. If you don't, you only make matters worse." (Ward Cleaver)

"The last of the human freedoms—to choose one's attitude in any given set of circumstances, to choose one's own way." (Viktor Frankl)

"Good people are good because they've come to wisdom through failure." (William Saroyan)

"I've had much to worry about—most of which did not happen." (Walt Whitman)

"Imagination is more important than knowledge." (Albert Einstein)

"Everything that irritates us about others can lead us to an understanding of ourselves." (Carl Jung)

"If I had a formula for bypassing trouble, I would not pass it round. Trouble creates a capacity to handle it. I don't embrace trouble; that's as bad as treating it as an enemy. But I do say meet it as a friend, for you'll see a lot of it and had better be on speaking terms with it." (Oliver Wendell Holmes)

"There is a miracle in every new beginning." (Hermann Hesse)

There will always be problems, challenges and stresses in our lives, because it is the nature of our work and of being human. As these quotes suggest, it is how we respond to these events that make a difference in our lives.

Katz's Work on the Hardy Dentist

Cliff Katz, a dentist and psychologist, has applied Suzanne Kobasa's work on the hardy person to dentistry. Kobasa found a cluster of personality factors in executives who were more resistant to stress. Kobasa labeled these people Hardy types. Kobasa found three general characteristics that these people shared. **Control:** The belief that they could control or influence the events in their life. **Commitment:** A deeply felt commitment to the institutions and activities in their lives. **Challenge:** The anticipation of change as an exciting challenge to further development.

```
CHALLENGE
COMMITMENT
CONTROL
```

Figure 8. The Three C's

Katz wrote a beautiful essay, "In Search of the Hardy Dentist." Katz's research in dentistry confirmed the findings of Kobasa. In his research, he related Hardiness to the level of perceived stress and career satisfaction in 300 randomly selected practicing dentists of the Texas Dental Association. The dentists who scored low on the Hardiness scale were more likely to rate dentistry as stressful and were less likely to feel satisfied with their choice of dentistry as a career.

Katz did a review of the literature on stress among dentists and found that many personality characteristics of dentists as a group contribute significantly to their stress levels. These researchers discussed the perfectionistic, high achiever, Type A, rigid, authoritarian, conservative and highly pragmatic characteristics of most dentists as predisposing these dentists to high levels of stress.

Paradoxically, many characteristics that have enabled these dentists to be successful in the technical aspects of dentistry are a hindrance in times of rapid change and in the presence of problems and frustrations. In times of turbulent change, these strengths become weaknesses. In turbulent times, Katz feels the personality characteristics of openness, flexibility and a high tolerance for ambiguity are more appropriate in coping with change. Katz states, "In other words, the degree of stress in dentistry appears not to be a function of characteristics of dentistry, but rather a function of the characteristics of the person who is practicing dentistry."

Katz's experience with dentists whom he would describe as hardy, leads him to believe that these people were not born this way, but they have learned to be hardy. He states, "Becoming Hardy is a process of growth and change that may take many forms, but always takes time and concerted effort."

There it is again the emphasis on learning, growth and change and creating conditions that support and facilitate positive change. The difference is that this time the emphasis is on creating these conditions for the caregiver, so he can heal his own woundedness.

When he is wounded the dentist needs to embark upon the hero's journey through the vale of tears, which trials and tribulations create, to heal himself.

Creating Healing Rituals

Rituals are usually seen as meaningless exercises or rules that are imposed from without and are discarded or are mindlessly done. When rituals come from within (remember de Chardin's quote) they are powerful enablers of change. To go through the vale of tears that the trials and tribulations of dentistry create, I feel it is important for the dentist to create healing rituals in his life. My definition of a ritual is an activity that when repeated often enough assumes a meaning of it's own, and creates meaningful change in one's life. Rituals are important facilitators of healing and give meaning to life transitions and events. The healing rituals cluster about nutrition, exercise, relationships, humor and play, positive focusing, knowing yourself and your personal history, creating meaningful work, honoring sacred moments, the ability to give and receive love, a belief in a higher power and professional counseling.

Nutrition—anything that nourishes. The root meaning of nutrition and nurture is the same "nutrire," to nourish. In respect to diet, nutrition is the science or study of a proper balanced diet to promote health. Dentists are well schooled in the importance of diet and health. What about the other things we take in? Do we surround ourselves with people who support and nurture us? Do we give as much time or more thinking about what is right in our lives as we do with what is wrong? Do we take time in our life to create through images what we want our life to be? Have we created external and internal environments that nourish us (home, office, gardens)? Does our dental practice nurture us?

Exercise—to put into action or employ. Traditionally, exercise is thought of as exercising the body as in the proper amount of aerobic exercise. Do you exercise your other aspects? Do you put into action your knowledge of what is good for you? Do you exercise your intellect, your creativity, your ability to learn? Do you put yourself in situations that are good for you and avoid situations that are destructive? Do you get the proper kind and amount of exercise food, and rest? Do you change negative thought patterns into a positive focus?

Relationships. As mentioned in other chapters, have you created healing relationships with others in your life? When you are troubled, are there people and groups in your life you can turn to for help?

Humor. Norman Cousins described laughter as internal jogging. Life is often so ridiculous that it should not be taken seriously. Is there an abundance of humor and joy in your life? Humor is healing if it is affectionate, spontaneous and warm. Do you engage in activities that make you laugh or bring you joy? Is one of these activities your dental practice? Who are the people in your life that you have fun with? Do you spend a significant amount of time with them? When life gets ridiculous, can you laugh at the absurdity of it all?

Play. All of us are childlike and love to play. Play gives us a chance at re-creation. "Play," Richard Cabot said, "keeps the soul alive." Katz's research on the Hardy dentist showed that the dentists that had balance in their life between work and play can cope better with stress. Often, dentist's leisure activities are as intense as their worklife. They carry their obsessions into their play on the tennis court, on the golf course, in the garden. Does your play revitalize you? Does it give a sense of re-creation?

Positive Focusing. Our thoughts, both positive and negative, are the most powerful determinants of the quality of our life. Thoughts are metaphysical energy that can drain us or enervate us. Rolling Thunder, an Indian medicine man said:

> *"People have to be responsible for their thoughts so they can learn to control them. It may not be easy but it can be done."*

He emphasized the importance of speaking with good purpose, and not paying attention to unwanted thoughts of continually making choices to think with clear and pure minds. He said "you can think what you choose—If they (unwanted thoughts) keep coming into your head, just let them alone and say, 'I don't choose to have such thoughts.'"

The theme of positive focusing, of focusing on what is right, what is good, true and beautiful, is common to all religions and cultures. It has been a difficult lesson for me to learn that I am responsible for my thoughts. Thoughts do not happen by accident. I can change them and by changing them, I determine the quality of my life. I can make my butterflies fly in formation.

Knowing yourself and your personal history. Socrates said it first, "Know yourself." Do you know what your stress buttons are? Do you know how your personal history—the schooling, family and personal events—has shaped you? Do you understand how these events are manifested in your life?

Most dentists are practicing or recovering perfectionists. This myth of perfection that is instilled in dentists in dental school (and by the way you were brought up), needs to be replaced with the recognition of the dentist's humanness. David Burns wrote that "Fear always lurks behind perfectionism. Confronting your fears and allowing yourself the right to be human can, paradoxically, make you a far happier and more productive person."

Knowing that your personal history from dental school and your family contributed to the unrealistic expectation of perfection and replacing it with more realistic expectations, is foundational to caring for yourself. Dentists are high achievers. They have successfully jumped over many hurdles on their way to becoming a dentist. Mistakes and failure are not handled well by most dentists and yet they happen. James Joyce said, "Mistakes are the portals of discovery." Knowing yourself and how you respond to events is important. This self-awareness is the beginning of changing destructive habits, beliefs and thought patterns—especially the myth of perfection.

Creating meaningful work. There is a difference between a job and a career or a profession. A job is something you do to earn money, to pay the bills and to enable you to do things you enjoy doing. A career or profession is work that you do because you enjoy it of and for itself. Noel Coward said, "Work is much more fun than fun."

One of the biggest stressors in dentistry is the perception of dentistry as a job. There was a time in my life when I physically shuddered as I contemplated going to the office or even as I drove by my office on weekends. Many dentists feel trapped by the income they derive from dentistry. They need the income from dentistry to support the things they enjoy doing. Or they feel so deep in debt that they cannot envision a way to leave dentistry or to do what they want to do in dentistry.

This brings us to the issue of money and the issue of how much is enough? Emmett Miller defines money as "stored human time and energy and as such it is a sacred trust and must be used wisely and for good." Money is a vehicle for placing a value on the life energy you invest in helping your clients to attain what they want. It is your attitude toward money that determines whether it will be a synergistic or destructive force in your life. It can be a great facilitator to live an enriching life, or it can be very destructive if we always feel as if there is not enough.

An important question is how much is enough? One of the Rockefellers replied to this question "Just a little bit more." This attitude is like a horse chasing a carrot on a stick and results in continual dissatisfaction.

I have come to value a life of voluntary simplicity. Duane Elgin defines Voluntary Simplicity as "a manner of living that is outwardly more simple and inwardly more rich: an integrative way of living that balances both the inner and outer aspects of our lives, a deliberate choice to live with less in the belief that more of life will be returned to us in the process."

The ability to give and receive love. Love is a heavily charged word and has many different meanings in different contexts. I like Hugh Prather's definition of love. "Love expands: it not only sees more and enfolds more, it causes its object to bloom. — We need other people, not in order to stay alive, but to be fully human: to be affectionate, funny, playful, to be genuine." Love is a belief in the basic goodness of life. The ability to give and receive love is the affirmation of our reason for being. It gives meaning and direction to our life. It is our connection with the divine and sacred, and it is how the divine and sacred are manifested in our lives.

Honoring Sacred Moments. There are many sacred moments in our lives. Times when we feel connected with the divine source in our lives. These moments can be noticed by the feelings of peace, joy, well being and love in our deepest being. Some examples of sacred moments are: watching a beautiful sunset, laughing with friends, a look or gesture of gratitude from a client or co-worker, meaningful walks or talks with your spouse, feeling "in the zone" when playing your favorite sport, meditation or prayer, watching animals, realizing the sacred nature of life, responding well to a situation that usually stresses you to your limits, a simple or complex procedure done well with a client. There are countless other examples of sacred moments. These moments happen frequently in our lives, yet we do not take the time to honor them, to appreciate them, to let them seep into our consciousness and permeate our sense of self worth. But give me a problem that hurts, bothers or worries me and watch the time I spend paying attention to the problem by dwelling on it and letting it consume my life by forcing out all other aspects of my life.

Recognizing the sacred moments in your life and honoring these moments by letting them fill your life with joy, peace and love, is the best work you will do in your life. Venerate sacred moments by spending more time in your life recognizing them, enjoying them, feeling them and letting them radiate throughout your life.

Belief in a Higher Power. Belief in the supernatural is common to all cultures. It has many forms: religion, spirituality, belief in the unknown mystery of life. This belief in a higher power, in the divine and sacred, sustains people through life's greatest trials and tribulations. Meditation, contemplation, quiet time and prayer are the common ways people connect with the divine and sacred. I have come to recognize that my career in dentistry is a spiritual journey and has aspects of the sacred and divine.

Professional Counseling. There are times when a part of caring for yourself involves asking for help from skilled empathic professional counselors, such as psychologists, psychotherapists, social workers or clergy members. These skilled counselors can serve as guides to help you gain understanding and perspective on the problems that are bothering or haunting you.

These healing rituals help caregivers restore and heal themselves on their life journey. They give meaning and direction to their personal and work life and enable them to help their clients heal.

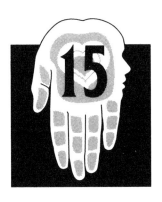

Dentistry as a
Spiritual Discipline,
A Return to the Sacred

Over the past few years, I have come to realize that for me dentistry has been a path of spiritual discipline and growth, that has resurrected in me a feeling of the sacredness in my life. Primarily, this recognition has come about from my experience in learning about the human dimensions of dentistry. This discipline of the spiritual life has had the hallmarks of the spiritual quest. Faith, doubt, self-realization, fear, enlightenment, transcendence, joy, peace, anxiousness, love, harmony, knowing and wholeness.

Before I write about my spiritual path in dentistry, I would like to write about my first experience with rites of initiation into a sacred time. Recently, I have had glimmers that somewhere in my past there was a time when I had gone through a spiritual experience. I could not put my finger on what the experience was until I attended a workshop on Imagery in Healing. During this workshop the presenters, Jeanne Acterberg and Frank Lawlis, used an Indian drum as part of an imaging exercise. The rhythms of the drum beat brought back memories of my initiation and experiences in the Tribe of Mic-O-Say. In retrospect, this was my initiation into the metaphysical world.

At the time, I would not have known what metaphysical meant, but I was filled with wonder, awe, a sense of magic and a realization of truths that had been beyond my understanding. The Tribe of Mic-O-Say is not an ancient Indian tribe that I was a part of in a past life, but an honorary organization based on Native American Indian traditions in the Kansas City Area Council of the Boy Scouts of America.

Rites of Initiation

So, through the memories of the years, I want to share my rites of initiation with you. These rites occurred when I was 14 years old. In traditional Indian times, 12–13 was when Indian children experienced similar rites. These rites included the initiate finding his sacred place and meditating for three to four days, while waiting for a vision that would give them a feeling to choose their name and their purpose in life.

In my third summer as a camper at Camp Osceola, I knew I might be called to the tribe. A ceremony named Call Night occurred. Call Night was a time of high suspense and drama for those who hoped to be called into the tribe. I sat in the stands outside the council ring, with the beat of the drums pounding in my ears, hoping to be called. The Chief called out the names of those who were called to become Foxman. I waited anxiously for my name to be called. The moment finally came; I was called. I came down into the council ring and was challenged by Medicine Man Lone Star—"Understand you, do you understand Foxman?"—to see if I understood the meaning of being called. I gave a frightened affirmative nod and he pushed me into the arms of a Runner. The runner ran me out of the council ring and I entered into a mystical three days of prayer, silence, meditation, contemplation, service, love, courage, fear, awe, altered consciousness and confusion. This experience remains one of the transcendent experiences of my life. As I write this, there are tears in my eyes and tingles in my body as these memories come rushing back.

This was a time of hard labor, rituals, secret ceremonies, drum beats, of being in nonordinary reality, of learning the customs and traditions of the Tribe of Mic-O-Say and contemplating my relationship with my family, community, and the world. The rites of initiation culminated in Lone Bear Council Ring as I and my fellow Foxman received the symbol of becoming a Tribesman.

I spent the next four summers as a staff member at Camp Osceola. I participated in initiating others into the Tribe and learned lessons of leadership, responsibility, integrity and organization. I was a teenager learning to be a warrior in the world.

My last year on staff was after my senior year in high school. That fall, I went to college and began my education to become a dentist. Looking back, I realize the lessons I learned at scout camp gradually receded as I learned about the scientific method, drugs, preparations, diagnosing, treating and curing. I lost the sense of the sacred, of my relationship with nature, my connection to my fellow human beings, my sense of wonder and awe at my place in the world. I lost the sense of sacred to the point that when I began another spiritual journey twenty years later, I had no memory of the lessons I had learned as a Tribesman. It took the beat of a drum to remind me of my first spiritual initiation.

Losing Contact

My education had pushed this sacred time into the background and had replaced it with an objective, agnostic rationality. Along with the influence of my education, I was very concerned in my early years in dentistry with financial and technical achievement. I did not place a high value on the human and spiritual dimensions of my life. Carl Jung stated that the first half of a person's life is devoted to external accomplishments, to developing ego, to achieving a sense of competence, while the last half of a person's life should be oriented to developing a sense of meaning in life, to an inward journey, to letting go of ego.

Recently, I have realized that dentistry has been a spiritual teacher for me. I have learned many spiritual lessons because of my interactions with my clients, colleagues and co-workers. These lessons have not been a result of formal rites of initiation as my initiations into the Tribe of Mic-O-Say were, but they have been because of my "practice" of dentistry.

Metaphysical Questions

In dental school, I learned about the systems of the body through courses in anatomy, biochemistry, physiology, bacteriology and histology. I also learned how to treat the malfunctions of these systems through pharmacology, surgery and restorative techniques. I learned that the body was an object and when it malfunctioned, it needed an objective cure through a drug, surgery, or rehabilitative technique. In my early years as a dentist, I did not question this mechanistic approach.

It was fifteen years later before I questioned this approach. At this time, a series of metaphysical questions passed through my mind, "What is it that gives life to this body? What gives animation, the life force to a person? Where does meaning come from? Why does a person want to be well? What are feelings for? Where does curiosity start? What creates love?" Why is a caring doctor-patient relationship so important in a client's healing?

When I asked these questions, when I looked at my clients and wondered about the life force that created this body, this mind, this spirit. In asking these questions, I met God.

The Role of Spirit

I simply had no rational explanation for the intangible aspects of my relationship with my clients and for what was the healing essence of their being. The role of spirit entered my professional life. How a person heals is truly a miracle. The body is injured through infection or trauma, and a process occurs to bring health, healing and wholeness back into the injured person's life. I could mechanically describe the process of the healing as the body's immune system responded to the injurious event. When a person experiences emotional trauma through a divorce, loss of a job or a spouse, they experience the dark night of the soul and begin the ascent toward light and life again. What led to the beginning of this process? There was a spirit that led to the healing, resurrection of health and well being.

What was that spirit? This recognition of spirit occurred in a cartoon that depicted a group of physicists coming out of their lab with bulging eyes saying, "You'll never guess who we just met." I was in awe of the role that I played in this healing process. I was the recipient of thousands of years of experience and knowledge of how to help people heal. The lives of past shamans, medicine men and women, priests, herbologists, and doctors had much more meaning for me as the spiritual dimension of healing dawned for me.

The Great Chain of Being

My experience in science had no answers to these questions. The Cartesian body-mind split was of no help to me in these areas. These were metaphysical questions that threw me into another spiritual quest similar to my youthful quest as a Foxman in the Tribe of Mic-O-Say. I don't have an answer to these questions and probably never will. Science will never completely answer these questions.

The perennial philosophers use the Great Chain of Being to describe the hierarchy of the spiritual path. The following diagram describes the Great Chain of Being.

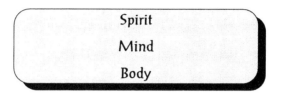

Figure 9. The Great Chain of Being

The body includes the lower level; the mind the middle level; and the spirit the higher level. In health care, we deal with the physical and biological aspects of the person and occasionally there are some doctors that include the mind and psychological aspects. Rarely are the spiritual aspects included in health care. The body is the densest and lowest layer of this hierarchy. The reductionistic model has been very effective in dealing with the physical aspects and the highest accomplishments of health care have occurred in this area. Drugs, surgery, and restorative techniques have been very successful in treating this physical area.

The reductionistic model works well at the physical level and has applicability at the biological level, but it is not as effective. Heart disease and cancer are good examples. The reductionistic model has not found a single causative agent for cancer and heart problems. Treatment for these diseases is much more complex, expensive, takes more time and is not as effective. The strengths of the reductionistic approach become less effective and even become weaknesses as we ascend the great chain of being.

Doctors are beginning to shed the dogma of reductionism and include other ways of helping people. The ungainly term psychoneuroimmunology (PNI) is used to describe a holistic approach to health care. PNI is a cluster of approaches that enables the client to mobilize their immune system to combat the precipitating event. These methods have been and are being developed for the biological and psychological levels. Imaging, exercise, relaxation exercises, biofeedback, humanistic psychotherapy, dream analysis and hypnosis are examples of holistic approaches that are used in treatment of mind-body problems, such as headaches, chronic pain, ulcers, heart problems, cancer, depression, burn out, stress management and emotional pain.

At the level of spirit, prayer and meditation are the most common approaches used to heal spiritually. There are many reports of so called "spontaneous remissions" in people who have been diagnosed with terminal cancer. These persons usually report a nonordinary event, (renewed sense of purpose, a vision, a reconciliation, change in relating with others etc.) as what they believe is the causative element.

Ken Wilber states, "that each level in the Great Chain transcends but includes its predecessor(s). That is each higher level contains functions, capacities, or structures not found on, or explainable solely in terms of, a lower level. The higher level does not violate the principles of the lower, it simply is not exclusively bound or explainable by them." (Wilber,1984).

There is research to support the concept of spiritual approaches that help heal. The work done by the Spindrift research group on yeast cultures showed that prayer works in controlling the proliferation of the yeast. This research showed that nondirected prayer was two to four times more effective than directed prayer.

A Sense of the Sacred

My recognition of the spiritual gave a sense of the sacred to my practice of dentistry. I began to sense that there was a spirit present in my work. Gerald May wrote that "Spiritual Practice always involves going beyond simply finding out who one is to a level of finding out also what one needs to do in the world." (May, Will and Spirit: A Contemplative Psychology, 1982, pp. 160–161). I sensed a new meaning behind the words human being and saw how they were related to each other. Human-being. There are two aspects of human beings; one is our humanness and one is our beingness. Life is a process of humans-being and of being-human. The part of our self that is being is our connection with the divine, with spirit. Our being is the way spirit is manifested through us. It is present to us always. When we are attuned to the spirit, we express the spirit in our actions, beliefs and behavior.

Our humanness is how we learn to manifest the spirit. In our humanness we make mistakes, we hurt ourselves and others. But our humanness is how we become divine. As we learn from our mistakes we come more in alignment with spirit. Our humanness is the vehicle in which we move from darkness to light. It is how we become enlightened.

These ideas are not new. They have existed for ages. In our times, they are "revolutionary old ideas." As health professionals have more experiences with the relational aspects of healing, which includes the spiritual, we will learn more about the foundational principles of healing and spirit and will be more able to facilitate healing in our clients, ourselves and our world. By learning to listen deeply to ourselves and our clients, we can listen to the divine and sacred spiritual source of our being.

Courage

Courage, with its attendant risks, ambiguity, joy, commitment and potential for transcendence, is necessary in ourselves and our clients to embark and keep upon the path toward this way of being. This healing doctor-patient relationship requires a different way of being together for the client and doctor. It goes far beyond the traditional doctor-patient relationship. It requires that both are active, responsible partners in the healing relationship; that both are vulnerable; that both are open to change in their lives; that both are open to the effects of these changes; that both use this courage to create a relationship in which both will take another step in the healing process.

Bibliography

* = recommended reading

Acterburg, Jeanne, *Imagery in Healing*. Boston, New Science Library, 1985.

Aspy, Roebuck, There is a beautiful summary in the chapter on "Researching person-centered issues in Education" in Roger's *Freedom to Learn for the 80's* of 19 articles on their research of person-centered approaches in education.

Avila, Combs, and Purkey ed. *The Helping Relationship Sourcebook*. 2nd edition, Boston: Allyn And Bacon, 1985.

Avila, Combs ed., *Perspectives on Helping Relationships and the Helping professions*. Boston: Allyn and Bacon, 1985.

* Barkley, Robert, *Successful Preventive Dental Practices*. Macomb, Illinois: 1972.

Benjamin, Alfred, *The Helping Interview*. Boston: Houghton Mifflin, 1969.

Boyd, Doug, *Rolling Thunder*. New York: Dell, 1974.

Campbell, Joseph, *The Power of Myth*. New York: Doubleday, 1988.

Carlisle, Lynn, "The Odyssey of Dr. Becoming." Nexus, 1977.

Carlisle, Lynn, "Dr. Becoming Revisited." Nexus, 1978.

Carlisle, Lynn, "Cracks/Transformation." Nexus, 1978.

Carlisle, Lynn, "Listening as a Part of Healing." *Healing Currents*, Vol. 10, No. 3 & 4, 1986.

Church, T., Moretti, R. and Ayer, W.A., "Issues and Concerns in the development of the dentist-patient relationship. New Dentistry, Vol. 10(7), 1980.

Combs, Avila, and Purkey, *Helping Relationships*. Boston: Allyn and Bacon, 1971.

Combs, Avila, *Helping Relationships*. 3rd edition. Boston: Allyn And Bacon, 1985.

* Combs, Arthur and Gonzalez, David M., *Helping Relationships*. 4th edition. Boston: Allyn and Bacon 1994.

Combs, Arthur, *A Personal Approach to Teaching*. Boston: Allyn and Bacon, 1985.

Combs, Arthur, *Myths in Education*. Boston: Allyn and Bacon, 1979.

Combs, Arthur, "What makes a Good Helper?" Person-Centered Review, Vol.1 No. 1 February 986, 51–61.

Cousins, Norman, *Human Options*. New York: W.W.Norton, 1981.

* Dossey, Larry, *Beyond Illness*. Boston: New Science, 1984.

* Egan, Gerard, *The Skilled Helper*. 2nd edition. Monterery, Ca.: Brooks Cole, 1982.

* Elgin, Duane, *Voluntary Simplicity*. New York: William Morrow, 1981.

Eron, L.D., "Effect of Medical Education on Medical Students Attitudes," Journal of Medical Education, Vol 30, 1955.

* Fischer and Ury, *Getting to Yes*. Boston: Houghton Mifflin, 1981.

* Fuller, Buckminster, *Critical Path*. New York: St. Martin's Press, 1982.

Gardiner, James F. and Sundin, Robert H., "Some principles of Communication at the dental Chairside," Journal of the Louisana Dental Association, Vol 34, Winter 1976.

Garity, Thomas F., "Medical Compliance and the Clinician-Patient relationship: A review. Social Science and Medicine 15E, 1981.

* Gordon, Thomas, *Teacher Effectiveness Training*. New York: Davis-McKay, 1974.

Inlander, Levin and Weiner, *Medicine On Trial*. New York: Prentice Hall, 1988.

Kamensky, Carol S., Museo, Laura, Naiman, Sandra, "Who's Killing the American Dentist?, Journal of the Colorado Dental Association, January/February 1986.

Kaplan, Sherrie H. and Greenfield, Sheldon, "Assessing the effects of physician-patient interactions in the outcomes of chronic disease." Journal of Medical Care Vol. 27 1989.

* Katz, Clifford, *In Search of the Hardy Dentist*. Nexus, Dec. 1981.

Kelley and Rasey, *Education and the Nature of Man*. 1952.

Lynch, James J., *The Language of the Heart*. New York: Basic Books, 1985.

* Maslow, Abraham, *Motivation and Personality*. New York: Harper and Row, 1970.

* Mayeroff, Milton, *On Caring*. New York: Harper Perennial, 1971.

Miller, Alice, *For Your Own Good*. New York: F.S.G., 1984.

* Pankey and Davis, *A Philosophy of the Practice of Dentistry*. Toledo, Ohio: Medical College Press, 1985.

* Prather, Hugh, *Notes to Myself*. Toronto: Bantam, 1970.

* Prather, Hugh, *Notes on Love and Courage*. Garden City, N.Y.: Doubleday, 1977.

Prigogine, Ilya, *From Being to Becoming*. San Francisco, Ca.: W.H. Freeman, 1980.

Polanyi and Prosch, *Meaning*. Chicago, Ill.: Chicago Press, 1975.

Remen, Naomi, *The Human Patient*. Garden City, N.Y.: Anchor Press, 1980.

Rogers, Carl, "A Note on the Nature of Man." Journal of Counseling Psychology, 1957.

* Rogers, Carl, *On Becoming a Person*. Boston: Houghton Mifflin, 1961.

Rogers, Carl, *Freedom to Learn*. Columbus, Ohio: Merrill, 1969.

Rogers, Carl, *On Personal Power*. New York: Dell, 1977.

Rogers, Carl, *A Way of Being*. Boston: Houghton Mifflin, 1980.

*Rogers, Carl, *Freedom to Learn for the 80's*. Columbus, Ohio: Merrill, 1983.

* Seigel, Bernie, *Love, Medicine and Miracles*. New York: Harper and Row, 1986.

Starr, Paul, *The Social Transformation of American Medicine*. New York: Basic Books, 1982.

Trungpa, Chogyam, *Shambhala*. Boulder: Shambhala, 1984.

* Vaughan, Frances, *Inward Arc*. Boston: Shambhala, 1985.

Whittemore, Burstein, Loucks, and Schoenfeld, "A Longitudinal Study of Personality Changes in Medical Students," Journal of Medical Education, Vol 59, October 1984.

Wilber, Ken, "Of Shadows and Symbols: Physics and Mysticism," Re Vison, Vol 7 No 1, 1984.

Wolf, Thomas M, and Kissling, Grace E., "Changes in Life-Style Characteristics, Health, and Mood of Freshman Medical Students," Journal of Medical Education, Vol 59, October 1984.

Index

NOTES

NOTES

NOTES

NOTES

NOTES

HOW TO CONTACT THE AUTHOR

Lynn D. Carlisle
373 West Drake Road
Ft. Collins, CO 80526

(970) 223-1420
(970) 223-1190 FAX

Available for
Consultations, Speaking Engagements and
Workshop/Study group facilitation

To Order *IN A SPIRIT OF CARING*

CONTACT: **Kendall/Hunt Publishing company**
4050 Westmark, PO Box 1840
Dubuque, IA 52004-1840
OR
Call 1-800-228-0810